THE SHADOW PRINCIPLE

Reconciliation with Our Hidden Side

THE SHADOW PRINCIPLE

Reconciliation with Our Hidden Side

RUEDIGER DAHLKE, M.D.

Translated by Simone Duxbury

SENTIENT PUBLICATIONS

First Sentient Publications edition 2025

Copyright © 2010 by Ruediger Dahlke

All rights reserved. This book, or parts thereof, may not be reproduced in any form without permission, except in the case of brief quotations embodied in critical articles and reviews.

A paperback original

Book design by Laura Waltje
Cover Design by Laura Waltje
Cover Illustration by Utagawa Hiroshige

Library of Congress Control Number: 2024949623
Publisher's Cataloging-in-Publication Data
Names: Dahlke, Ruediger, author. | Duxbery, Simone, translator.

Title: The shadow principle : reconciliation with our hidden side / Ruediger Dahlke; translated by Simone Duxbery.

Description: Boulder, CO: Sentient Publications, 2025.

Identifiers: LCCN: 2024949623 | ISBN: 978-1-59181-346-0 (paperback) | 978-1-59181-347-7 (epub)
Subjects: LCSH Mind and body. | Shadow (Psychoanalysis) | Holism. | Holistic medicine. | Self-actualization (Psychology) | Jungian psychology. | Self-help. | MEDICAL / Holistic Medicine | MEDICAL / Alternative & Complementary Medicine | BISAC BODY, MIND & SPIRIT / Healing / General | PSYCHOLOGY / Psychotherapy / Jungian | HEALTH & FITNESS / Holism | SELF-HELP / Meditations
Classification: LCC BF175.5.S55 .D34 2025 | DDC 150.19/54--dc23

SENTIENT PUBLICATIONS
A Limited Liability Company
PO Box 1851
Boulder, CO 80306
www.sentientpublications.com

For suggestions and corrections, I would like to thank the long-standing staff and companions at the Heil-Kunde-Zentrum in Johanniskirchen: Christa Maleri, Anja Schönfuss, Hildegunde Kirkovics and Freda Jeske. I would also like to thank Dorothea Neumayr and Balthasar Wanz for their dedicated commitment. To my long-standing companion on the publishing side, Gerhard Riemann, I owe the encouragement to write this book and his contribution to its content; my thanks also go to Usha Swamy and Christine Stecher for their proven support on the publishing side. A big thank you goes to Bruce Weber and Claudia Fried for the music they provide in my professional life and their trusted collaboration, as well as to our secretary of many years at the Heil-Kunde-Zentrum, Rita Pichlmaier, for her support on the computer. For rearranging the order of the book, personal shadow work on me and numerous shadow-critical suggestions, I thank my most personal shadow and greatest treasure, my partner Rita Fasel.

Contents

A travel guide for the riches of the Shadow kingdom

Learning from your own perspective

Reconciliation with your own shadow kingdom is the most paramount, and at the same time, most fundamental goal that a person can set—and positing it as a goal for this book means that the aim is being set very high. As a result, this book is not a simple text for reading in the traditional sense, but more a journey into the shadow kingdom, with stops for practical training exercises along the way. It would therefore be *wonder*-ful and important for you, in addition to reading the text,

- to keep a shadow diary from the very beginning. This should be used to record the results of the questions and tests along the way, as well as the experiences gathered in the meditations and practical exercises.
- The accompanying meditations offers further practical possibilities for accessing the image world of the soul. The technique of guided meditation which it uses is very simple and leads to an impressive expansion of consciousness. You would simply need to complete the respective inner journey at the relevant

point in the book. This acts as an ideal complement to the diary. While the book helps you to wise up to the tricks of the shadow using investigative techniques and refinements that are similar to those of a famous detective like Sherlock Holmes, the guided journeys of the meditations fulfil the role of a Dr Watson, his investigative side-kick. Although less clever in an intellectual sense, Watson is nevertheless all the more intuitive and emotionally aware, and as a result, provides valuable input that stems from the heart and from gut feelings instead.

- The suggestions that are scattered throughout the book regarding certain (feature) films that it would be useful to watch on DVD at home bring light and shadow images from the external world into play. These are then connected in the practical exercises that follow to a whole that is more than the sum of its parts.

To put it in another way, the journey into the shadow world should ideally take place on various levels: for example, on the level of reading and understanding, but also on the experiential level when working through the various questions, suggested practical exercises, rituals, meditations and film meditations, and through the connection of all of these in a shadow diary. In this way, the latter should eventually become your own private book about shadow. Best of all would be if, over time, the process of reading itself would be enough to conjure up inner images that could be explored more deeply during the mind-imagery excursions in the meditations.

In short, the overall goal is to track down your own shadow, to come to terms with it, confront it and then eventually learn to accept it, in the sense of learning to love it. Since this is more a program rather than just a book, and in some stretches, even akin to therapy, you won't always be sent along strictly logical paths. In contrast, you will find that when travelling along the shadow path, theory and practice intentionally merge and mix together. For this reason, the book is not appropriate as a quick and easy read. You will benefit more from picking it up again and again. You have plenty of time—your whole life in fact—with or without the book, with or without therapy.

This book could be a good one to keep close at hand on your nightstand. When the shadow of nightfall descends upon us, it represents a very opportune time to voluntarily confront our shadow. This will in turn bring increasingly more light into our life and with it also more joy. Over time, you will even start to find it more and more fun to shine more light little by little into your own darkness, and in doing so, to become more conscious, broad-minded, open and friendly—towards others, but most of all, towards yourself. The shadow journey is, without a doubt, the most exciting adventure that we can undertake, and this book may be able to serve as a travel guide in keeping with the motto—"This above all: To thine own self be true."[1]

What is actually meant by the term "Shadow"?

Shadow is the unknown that makes us fearful. Even though it is often painted black, it conceals the entrance to everything that is light within us and to the light that is required by every form of greater consciousness, particularly so, by en*light*enment itself. In this respect, our shadow is actually the true key to life, although it is typically defamed as being darkness and evil. For C.G. Jung—the father of shadow psychotherapy—the shadow is the entire Unconscious. Basically, all symptoms—be they physical, emotional or psychological, or stemming from our social environment—are an expression of shadow.

Writing this book on shadow has made it clear to me how the lion's share of my books have been related to this topic. In

1 Shakespeare, *Hamlet*, Act 1, Scene III, l.78

effect, I spent close to thirty years working for the most part as a shadow therapist and have undergone quite a lot of shadow therapy myself. Nevertheless, as this book shows, I also seem not to have worked through the topic to a point of closure. The various shadow topics continue to accompany me, and you, as my audience, allow me to become conscious of them, which I would like to take this opportunity to thank you for. If, for example, at one of my talks, there is a large book table, many think to themselves and others voice openly, "He just can't get enough, can he?". If there is no book table, those same people say, "So now, he thinks he's too good to be selling books." Or "Probably he's already earned enough." Others upon seeing the many books on display think to themselves and then say out loud "Wow, he's really conscientious." They admire the work I've put into them and approach me to discuss it. If there is no book table, these people tend to have thoughts like, "He seems to be really modest. He doesn't even show his books openly." For the latter group, their shadow topic is their own creativity and modesty, and these are the topics they need to work on. For those mentioned earlier, it is their own financial problems and business savvy that are in shadow. For those people, I wrote the book *The Psychology of Money*. Both groups have something to do with me.

In addition to comparatively harmless symptoms and minor slip-ups as an expression of shadow topics, such as miserliness or shyness, we all know of more drastic examples for the outbreak of shadow in everyday life that are all the more terrifying because they are so unexpected and violent. A typical story in this respect: when it comes to Mr B., the ever-friendly and devoted family father, who has never hurt anyone in his life, everyone is used to him always putting his own interests last. Regarded by relatives and neighbours as exceptionally helpful, it is not uncommon for him to serve as a role model for others. Everyone is full of praise. He is the paragon of virtue, the model father, who sacrifices everything for his family, friends and colleagues. If you ask him for a favour, it is as good as guaranteed that he will satisfy your request. But one day, completely unexpectedly for everyone, he loses it and slips out of the role. For a brief moment, he becomes someone that no-one had known about until then: a violent perpetrator, who rams a bread knife into his wife and then chases after his son with murderous intent. As unexpectedly as it broke free, the demon vanishes. Mr B. now crumples into a small heap as it were—a picture of misery—and lets himself be taken into custody by the police without a hint of resistance. A journalist who later makes the vain attempt to put the "inexplicable" into words will describe him as a "broken man". One minute of dominance by the shadow has extinguished decades of well-organized, middle-class life. From one moment to the next, the good father has become the evil "shadow man" for everyone. It is with good reason that our world quickly forgets such "shadow men", banishing them as rapidly as possible from everyday life and putting them away in prisons or other institutions under lock and key.

For such extreme outbursts of shadow, the term "running amok" is now commonly used. Of Malayan origin, literally translated it means "to kill in blind rage". Interestingly, in earlier times in Asia, for example in Bali, the crime of running amok was not even punished. It was assumed that the people concerned were "beside themselves" and consequently were not responsible for their actions. In a certain way, this is even a modern view, as the discussion of split personalities (from pg 168 onwards) will later show. When the shadow has been consistently repressed over a long period, it can seem totally foreign to a person's nature, as if not belonging at all to that particular person.

The following medical "case history" provides a further example of the breaking through of shadow: a young patient, the father of two small children receives the diagnosis of testicular cancer in an advanced stage. The prognosis of the doctors is that he has one year to live at the most. Desperately, the man looks for a way out: If he worked like crazy, how much could he still manage to pay off on the mortgage of the semi-detached house that they have just moved into? How can he ensure that his family will be adequately provided for after he is gone? He is unable to find any solution. During a long discussion with the patient, my suggestion that he try taking up the fight for his life is more or less drowned out by the pessimistic tone being spread by the authoritative voice of conventional medicine. The "solution" that the patient then finds also takes me completely by surprise: since he cannot provide adequately for his family and can no longer save himself, he decides to fulfil an old dream of taking a trip around the world, which he had sacrificed when his wife became pregnant with their first child. He uses a small portion of the remaining money; the rest he leaves for his family. When he finally reaches his end and the debilitating weakness predicted by the doctors overwhelms him, he will seek a fitting place to die. Instead of psychotherapy, or in other words, an inner journey of the soul, he now wants tips for a trip in the outer world. Those he leaves behind respond with shock and outrage. The devastated wife who sent him to me in the first place now believes that she obviously never really knew her husband. He had never been inconsiderate and egotistical up to that point. Nevertheless, she does remember how eager he had been to go with her on a trip around the world and how they had abandoned the idea because of the pregnancy. They had gotten married instead and had had another child soon after, and he had started working straightaway instead of studying. In the course of the conversation, it becomes clear how welcome the pregnancy had been for her and how inopportune for him. It had spared her from having to overcome her fear of the world and had saved her from having to bear the uncertainty of their life situation at that point any longer. That, in keeping with her greatest wish, he would marry her, was something that she had known or at least hoped for. For him, the first child had taken away his freedom and the dream of a big, wide world, as well as the chance to study far away from home.

Both stories have something in common. In the case of running amok or developing cancer, shadow breaks through into everyday life and changes it radically. In contrast to the first story, which leads to a hopeless end in prison and defies explanation, the second has an unexpected ending. Half a year later, the young man is not weaker as predicted by the doctors, but instead is easily able to continue travelling. At the end of the year, he has long since reached the special place in India that he had chosen to die in, but while his money runs out, his life energy does not. He manages to scrape by and returns after almost two years away with no signs of the cancer. Later, his wife even takes him back.

Nowadays, I would say that the young man carried out a considerable portion of shadow work under his own direction and allowed a part of himself to live freely that had been repressed up to that point. His cancer was an outbreak of dark shadow, his breaking out on his own a breakthrough for light shadow. Both, however, were shadow aspects because they were unconscious. As soon as the patient willingly chose to devote energy to the shadow, the shadow was then able to give him the gift of so much strength and dynamic energy that he was able—without additional effort and without therapy—to defeat the cancer. This was something that the young man had definitely not expected. Upon his return, he was also not the same person he was when he had first headed off. His wife had been right: the part of him that had caused him to break off everything and break out on a whim was a part that she had never known. Probably he had hardly known that part of himself up till then either. The hopelessness of the cancer diagnosis had given him the strength to once again acknowledge the dream that he had banished to the shadows. By the time he returned, this part of himself had been allowed to live freely and had become integrated, making his life richer and more well-rounded for him and his family. Filled with this new energy, he began his course of studies.

Both examples show that the shadow invisibly casts its influence from our Unconscious. Nevertheless, in doing so, it can become the signpost for what is missing for us to become whole again. For this reason, our shadow is valuable and is, in fact, our greatest treasure. Admittedly, by definition, we do not "know" our shadow, but despite this, a journey into the shadow realm—as indicated by the second story—is enticing and full of wonderful possibilities. When we have the courage to head into new and unknown territory, it will inspire us and yield far more than taking the same trip to the same place over and over.

Shadow diary

Do I tend to travel to the same places for my vacation or do I feel drawn to unknown new territory? What could I resolve to do differently for my next vacation? Do I move around in life or do I tend to stay in the same place?

Note your thoughts.

Devils, demons and the "inner boarhound"

Shadow has been given many names in the course of history, both profound names and superficial ones. Regardless of these, shadow has always maintained its central and dominating role in life, even in times when we wanted to have nothing to do with it, as is the case in these modern times. In the Middle Ages, people referred to it as the inner demon, and those who devoted their attention to it assumed that they were "*wrestling with the devil*". Those who claimed "*the devil made me do it*" believed they had fallen under the influence of the shadow.

The confrontation with one's own demons is familiar to members of the clergy, as they have had to repress so much of their essential being, in particular, so many natural drives. However, these drives ended up driving them, and what was repressed ended up pressing upon their souls. The more they saw these demons as separate from themselves, the easier it was to shirk responsibility for their own dark side. As a result, they preferred to let the devil take the rap than to take responsibility for these drives themselves.

The demonization of others, the foisting of all kinds of blame or responsibility onto others is referred to by psychologists as "projection" (lat. *proicere* = to throw out, throw forward, throw forth). Nevertheless, it does not lead to a solution. On the contrary, it instead makes the topic that has been repelled and pushed away stronger and stronger until it eventually dominates that person's life. In this way, the devil as a classic shadow figure is always assigned a dominating role in the life of each individual, or indeed of a whole epoch, if aspects that are particularly important for life have been withdrawn from it and pushed onto the devil instead. Projection is thus the direct path to the creation of shadow.

To what extent even love that has been banished to the shadows can become a problem is shown by the example of Christianity—the religion of love. Its priests, who are forbidden to engage in the earthly, physical aspects of love and who are only allowed to feel love for the divine, have throughout history plummeted into the deepest depths of shadow in this respect. During the Inquisition, love took on its most perverted form in the guise of a clerical sadism that was responsible for the torturing to death of between one to nine million people, most of them women. Their deaths resulted from the clergy's battle against feminine attraction, the healing powers of older and wiser women and the pre-existing fertility-based religions. The main crime of these "witches" consisted in being attractive and in being healers who were able to regulate fertility. However, what actually happened in reality was that the masculine pole in the form of the male members of the clergy tried to slaughter their own feminine shadow in the form of the accused women—instead of integrating their own anima in the sense of C.G. Jung and thereby becoming more open and broad-minded towards their own feminine side in terms of empathy, sensuality, fertility and healing (becoming whole). The perverse logic of projection has probably never been made so terrifyingly clear as in this instance.

These clergymen could not imagine that the mere appearance of a woman could be enough to arouse a priest who had the blessing of God; she had to be in league with the devil. When they tortured her to death in orgies of torment that were as lecherous as they were sadistic, they were also saving her soul from the devil. In addition, it was much easier to bear the burden of celibacy if you allowed all of the attractive women in the area to be killed off, at the same time pocketed ninety percent of their possessions and then used the remaining ten percent to motivate and reward those who denounced these women in the first place. In direct comparison, the modern-day orgies of sexual abuse seem relatively harmless, but these are also an expression of the repressed shadow of human love that is not allowed the chance to exist in celibacy. The highest ideal in the form of divine love does not seem to properly satisfy many human priests and so they slip back down to the physical sexual level again and again, and on that level, to the most unredeemed and perverse variants of it. Despite this, it is actually love that is required, and particularly so of priests, who are the representatives of God's love on Earth. However, that love was never supposed to be as physically violent, as in the abominable Inquisition proceedings, nor as unsavoury as in the modern cases of sexual abuse. At the same time, it would be making things too easy if we simply projected onto the Church and its priests. Wherever there is a lot of light, there is also a lot of shadow. The history of Christianity has demonstrated that from its very beginnings. To put it another way, wherever there is a lot of shadow, there must also be a lot of light, for instance, in the form of all those priests who have not done anything wrong, but who are nowadays automatically reviled and vilified along with the others.

The fact that the Church finds it so difficult to engage in honest shadow therapy can show us just how difficult it is in general. At the same time, what a great chance for redemption it would be if, after a radical clean-up, the energy of clarification and renewal were granted enough space to allow a breath of fresh air to penetrate old walls and minds. Just how much energy could be set free by an honest plea for forgiveness and the openly-declared intention to make amends, especially if these were to be issued from the highest levels! In actual fact, the Church which, after all, is the last remaining refuge for the values of our culture is being called upon to carry out shadow therapy with the resultant reformation from the ground up. It would be the perfect opportunity to reform an oath like celibacy that is untenable in every respect, and which—despite the best intentions—has invoked so much shadow or unholy misery. This is especially the case given that it only has anything to do with Christ and his wonderful teachings about love to the extent that it has called up its darkest shadow.

Christ knew incidentally what he was doing when he built his church upon Peter, who already in the first night would betray him three times to save his own skin.[2] What the great master was willing to accept is something that modern-day Christians might find disconcerting. Nevertheless, knowledge of the overall pattern and the master plan could restore peace after a thorough process of reformation and shadow confrontation has taken place. Without being able to formulate it in such concrete terms, several million Catholic Christians are now sensing and demanding the necessity of doing this. Compared with this topic which resonates strongly with many of us, there are other topics, which are much easier to deal with. However, wherever shadow comes into play, it quickly becomes hard and unpleasant, particularly in those aspects where it is of personal significance to us.

Even as a demon, the shadow has seen better times. In Greek Antiquity, the Daimonion stood for the divine, and Socrates used this label for the highest, most divine part of the soul,

---

2 See the chapter "The Law of Beginnings" on this topic in my book *Die Schicksalsgesetze* (*The Laws of Fate*); Book overview available at www.dahlke.at/buecherliste

comparable with modern-day expressions, such as our conscience or inner voice, which we should listen to and obey.

In the antique sagas, the mythical heroes have to descend into the Underworld, for example, Heracles, who has to wrestle with Cerberus, the multi-headed "hound of Hades" guarding the entrance to the gates of Hell. In the German language, this dog is better known nowadays as "der innere Schweinehund" (literally: the inner boarhound). In English, we refer to this concept more commonly as our "inner demon", a trusted companion for substance addicts and anyone trapped in other unwanted forms of dependency. Anyone who looks carefully will find the inner demon in themselves. On the one hand, it allows us do things that we actually do not want to do. On the other hand, it gets in the way of us doing things that we want to do and should do, and that we, for example, consider to be healthy. We cast the blame for our failings onto our demon. For example, our demon gets the blame when we do not manage to go jogging, and this is also a form of projection: the casting off of responsibility. The truth, of course, is that our "inner boarhound" or our "inner demon"—nomen ist omen—is a part of us, a typical shadow aspect. We simply have very little contact to this other "will", and thus to a certain extent, feel like we are being controlled by an external force, as is typical for addictive behaviour. Whenever we shift the blame to someone else, projection, and with it once again, the topic of shadow is at play.

The battle of human heroes with this animalistic or dark counterpole is a classic confrontation with the shadow that runs through the mythical folklore of many different cultures. Siegfried, in doing battle with the dragon Fafnir, was the representative for many young heroes. The various heroic sagas and myths all tell us about how courageous warriors freed themselves and their country from evil monsters who were threatening to stifle all of life itself. These heroes grow beyond themselves, and by slaying the dragon, conquer their own shadow. After that, they can bring themselves and their country back to life. In this respect, these heroes stand for all of us, who in battling with our own shadow dragon, have so much to gain. We have to find our personal dragon, then corner it and finally confront it. By doing so, we have already more or less conquered it. In Chinese symbolism, the dragon has always been a symbol of good fortune right from the start. In our culture, we first have to make it to one. This is possible when we conquer it, by confronting our own darkness—the shadow world—and in this way, succeed in integrating it as a conscious aspect of ourselves. As a symbol for this, Siegfried bathes in the blood of the dragon, whereby all of the skin that is wet by it, becomes immune to the forces of destruction.

Even in the oldest sagas known to man, this motif can be recognized yet again: the Babylonian hero Gilgamesh, after winning the battle against his dark brother Enkidu, ends up gaining him as his strongest ally—a further indication of the great gifts that await us in the shadow kingdom.

The degree of honesty and authenticity that is necessary for this battle with the shadow is betrayed by another myth from Mesopotamia. In this one, the divine goddess Inanna in descending to face her dark antagonist—the goddess of the Underworld—has to confront her naked and without her symbols of grandeur. In other words, in the confrontation with her own dark side, she has to drop all masks.

All cultures know the shadow and describe it in their own way. Further names for the shadow are the dark twin, our double or doppelganger, the dark side, or for Freud, the Id. Following C.G. Jung, psychotherapists speak simply of the "shadow". From Jung we learn that the shadow is actually our greatest source of inspiration und offers the chance to find our way back to our spiritual roots. It can lead us far above the personality or person(a)—that mask, through which the conscious ego that we identify ourselves with (Latin *per* = through, *sonare* = to sound) resounds in the world. Jung regarded the shadow as the being that that we fear, that we would rather not be, but in the end, have to become, if we want to become one with everything. In this respect, shadow is extremely dichotomous. It repels us and tempts us closer; it disgusts us and fascinates us at the same time.

Jung also makes a further distinction between our personal shadow and the collective shadow. Our personal shadow arises through the suppression of characteristics that we would prefer not to identify ourselves with and that we do not want to accept, but that we nevertheless have.

It is from the collection of these suppressed characteristics that our shadow develops, and naturally, it grows over the course of our lives if we do not consciously intervene. It operates—unconsciously—behind our backs, and more often than not, makes a mockery of our conscious personality. In addition to the personal shadow that we will devote our attention to in the next chapters, the collective shadow comprises the unconscious topics of a culture or society, while the archaic shadow confronts us with our most primal fears.

Shadow diary

Is there something in my life that is getting in the way of satisfaction, good health and happiness?

Note your thoughts.

Repressing the shadow

Robert Bly, the author of *Iron John*[3], a book that deals, among other things, with the dark, masculine side, talks of the shadow as a sack that we drag behind us. Bly believes that, up to adolescence, or up to the point of becoming an adult, we are busy stuffing things into this black shadow sack that we are not willing to "bear" in our consciousness. We then spend the rest of our lives struggling to get those aspects of our soul back out of the sack and to integrate them into our lives. With

3 Robert Bly: *Iron John. A Book about Men.* Rider, New Edn, 2001

this metaphor, Bly offers a good summary of how shadow develops. During our childhood, youth and adolescence, we create shadow in order to develop our personality and to ensure our spiritual survival. When, as adults, we want to develop in the direction of self-actualization, we need to retrieve the content that has been pushed into the shadow and allow it to once again play a part in our lives.

The temptation to leave the cudgel in the sack and to fearfully ignore our unloved/unlived aspects is substantial. On the other hand, even children know that, in addition to the big stick and cudgel, St Nicolaus also has a lot of gifts in his big sack. Freeing these from the dark (shadow) sack is the task of this book and the most important one with respect to self-fulfilment. A life with the cudgel left in the sack becomes rather monotonous and boring. It does not so much peter out into quicksand as into the shadows, and the people concerned do not even notice it. In addition, they live with the constant threat of sudden outbreaks of shadow as shown by the stories that were recounted at the beginning of this chapter.

People who want to ignore the shadow resist the interpretation of symptoms, for example, illness patterns that enable shadow topics to come to light and to our awareness. In this way, the meaning of illness patterns is often embarrassingly obvious and—particularly for outside observers—impossible to overlook. Nevertheless, those affected prefer to deny the obvious in a childish way, and to deny the reality that is being shown in the symptom. That is why everyone else is spontaneously able to grasp what is going on, except for the person affected. Large sections of the population of modern industrialized countries have barricaded themselves into this situation in keeping with the motto: "Just don't stir things up".

In connection with this, the following provides a further example for the outbreak of shadow: an abbess, who had performed her monastic duties in an exemplary way over decades and who had always set a good example for her fellow sisters in every respect, suffered a dramatic outbreak of shadow, which those around her interpreted as a form of possession (by the devil). As psychiatrists, we just as obviously assumed it to be a form of psychosis. According to her fellow sisters, the afflicted woman had, without any prior warning, suddenly begun to strip off her clothing, to use rude and coarse words in a sexual context, to masturbate continually in public and to write alarming slogans on the wall of her cell using her own urine and faeces. The energy behind this outbreak of shadow was so powerful that even the strongest neuroleptic drugs (medication with a dampening effect in the treatment of psychoses) was scarcely able to deter her from it.

If, as a result of the repression strategy, the shadow becomes too massive, it can take over control and push the ego aside. In the past, people naturally spoke of possession and suspected the devil and demons to be behind it. In the era of the great psychiatrists Bleuler and Jung, the term dementia praecox (premature dementia) was used, thereby naming the shadow phenomenon according to its end stage. Nowadays, we very "scientifically" speak of schizophrenia—or of a psychosis if the shadow outbreaks occur only over a limit period of time. In addition to the shadow outbreaks mentioned at the beginning of the chapter in the sense of running amok and serious illness, psychosis represents a further unconscious confrontation with one's own dark side.

Only a few people are aware that, even in today's world, which has been put so cleanly in order and carefully freed of demons and superstition, a third of the population still falls victim to a psychosis at least once in their lifetime and thus to the shadow. More than a third of those afflicted manage to put this behind them as a one-off shadow experience, albeit perhaps one lasting several months. A further third continues to face frequent battles with such outbreaks from that point on, and just under a third ends up joined forever with the shadow in the sense of schizophrenia. This word describes a permanent psychological split (Greek: *schizein* = to split, *phren* = mind, soul). In other words, the connection between the ego and the shadow breaks off completely. Both go their separate ways, so to speak, and are no longer able to peacefully find their way back to each other.

Normally, in humans, the ego or the personality is at the helm and the shadow is repressed. It is only in illness symptoms or other symptoms—for example addictions, slip-ups, accidents or nightmares—that the shadow is able to make its presence felt in small ways. In contrast, for schizophrenics, it is the shadow that is in power and the ego that is repressed. The latter can only show itself in so-called "islands of clarity"[4], small moments of clear perspective. With the use of neuroleptic medication, psychiatrists try to suppress the shadow's means of expression—the hearing of voices and the flood of images—in order to give the ego a fighting chance and to strengthen it in the long term. Unfortunately, however, neuroleptics weaken the ego considerably. In contrast, shadow therapy, in the sense of this book tries to not let the shadow become so threateningly powerful in the first place, but instead to allow it to express itself before it is too late.

From the shadow side to the sunny side

The previously-mentioned figures regarding the frequency of psychoses indicate how great the shadow of our modern society actually is. Lately, shadow has suffered the same fate as the discipline that is responsible for taking care of it, namely the field of psychiatry. Both are similarly heavily laden with taboos and have been driven away to the outer fringes of society.

4 The concept stems from the American psychiatrist Edward M. Podvoll. His book *Recovering sanity. A compassionate approach to understanding and treating psychosis.* Boston: Shambhal. (2003) is highly recommendable.

When the shadow forces its way into consciousness, shoving the ego aside, it often feels to those afflicted like an invasion by a foreign power, with whom there are no opportunities for cooperation. This scenario of the largely-repressed shadow suggests that it would be better to arrange for a conscious and planned confrontation with one's shadow in the sense of therapy. Those who listen to their inner voice right from the start, which is what the practical exercises and meditations in this book encourage you to do, can feel comparatively safer from the forced entry of inner voices in the sense of psychiatry. Similarly, those who deal with their inner images in a relaxed way—both the images in their dreams and those on their guided journeys inward- can feel safer from the forced entry of overwhelming hallucinations.

The decision to let the cudgel out of the sack, or in other words, out of its hiding place in the form of the unconscious is difficult. It requires the overcoming of resistance, the fear of the shadow is just as massive as the knowledge of the gifts and treasures that are hidden within it is incredibly scant. In mythology, it is no coincidence that Pluto is both the god of the Underworld and the god of Wealth and Treasure. For enlightened people and those who would like to become so, the decision to devote oneself to one's shadow, despite all of its associated problems, is simply unavoidable. All of the religions and myths of the world are surprisingly unanimous in this respect: the way to the light always and only leads through the shadow. Even Christ had to descend into the realm of the dead before being resurrected on the third day.

As a rule, the everyday healthy normal citizen experiences shadow in a far less dramatic way and to a greater or lesser degree in the form of small blunders, such as Freudian slips, more harmless symptoms, and above all, in avoidance strategies. All of these already provide indications regarding our own unconscious domain. When it comes to people in the spotlight or those who have high ethical standards and a position of great responsibility, every example of the eruption of shadow, such as going off the rails sexually, the consumption of drugs or the breaking of other societal taboos, give the press reason to rejoice about the fact that they can then drag these into the spotlight of public attention. An example of this is the highly-regarded protestant bishop Margot Käßmann, who one night got drunk and drove through a red light straight into the arms of the police. With as much surprise and shock as the woman herself, the public wondered how something like that could happen to her of all people.

Pursuing such shadow experiences in this book is, on the one hand, a form of preventative measure. The process aims at rendering such extreme outbreaks of shadow, which we would then be helplessly at the mercy of, superfluous. On the other hand, it is also designed to enrich one's life to a degree that is scarcely imaginable, and does so by integrating unconscious aspects that make us fearful.

Whereas St Nicolas only comes once a year with his giant sack inclusive big stick and presents, our shadow is always with us, and can reward or punish us on a daily basis. The decision is ours. Those who choose to look inside the sack to take advantage of the presents will find a wealth of material in this book and its practical exercises. This will also make the use of the big stick unnecessary.

A very inspiring example for the reversal in polarity from the shadow to the light or sunny side is conveyed by the text of the Lost Generation by Jonathan Reed, which won him a prize at the 2006 Cannes Lions International Festival of Creativity (see below). Read in the traditional sequence from top to bottom, it describes with terrible bluntness the depressing situation of the youth of today in our modern world. Reading it line for line from bottom to top and from thought grouping to thought grouping, the same text transforms into a revelation regarding a better future. This clever palindrome can be viewed at https://www.youtube.com/watch?v=42E2fAWM6rA

- I am part of a lost generation
- and I refuse to believe that
- I can change the world
- I realize this may be a shock but

- »Happiness comes from within.«
- is a lie, and
- »Money will make me happy.«
- So in 30 years I will tell my children
- they are not the most important thing in my life
- My employer will know that
- I have my priorities straight because
- work
- is more important than
- family
- I tell you this
- Once upon a time
- Families stayed together
- but this will not be true in my era
- this is a quick fix society
- Experts tell me
- 30 years from now, I will be celebrating the 10th anniversary of my divorce
- I do not concede that
- I will live in a country of my own making
- In the future
- Environmental destruction will be the norm
- No longer can it be said that
- my peers and I care about this earth
- It will be evident that
- my generation is apathetic and lethargic
- It is foolish to presume that
- There is hope.

And all of this will come true
unless we choose to **reverse it.**

The astonishment at this reversal, which is equally as simple as it is effective, is a wonderful accompaniment on our journey through the shadow to the light. Later we will indeed do exactly that, and will learn in our most important shadow game of all to make friends out of enemies and to extract light from shadow.

The Darkness in Everyone —

Coming to terms with polarity

In our confrontation with our shadow, our breathing reveals the problem, but at the time, also the solution. We do not judge breathing out or breathing in; we value both poles and consider both of them to be important. We do not favour one pole or the other, and the rhythm of our breathing carries us consistently and safely through life—as long as we maintain this balanced appraisal of the situation.

Rhythm arises from the constant alternation between two poles and is essential for life. Rudolf Steiner, the founder of anthroposophy, was of the opinion that all life itself is nothing but rhythm. It is certainly true that life unfolds in the world of opposites through the rhythmic interplay between poles, which is not only evident in our breathing. If we bring judgement into play (in the game of life), problems develop immediately. For example, if we prefer the taking aspect of breathing in more than the giving aspect of breathing out, a life-threatening problem develops straightaway. By preferring breathing in, breathing out sinks into the shadow realm—the situation in bronchial asthma. A preference for breathing in automatically disadvantages breathing out. Those afflicted struggle and gasp desperately for air, but in their desperation, forget to breathe out as well. For many asthmatics, this mistake even eventually proves fatal.

This example illustrates an important mechanism of shadow formation. Any time we reject something—in this case breathing out and giving—it does not simply disappear, but instead sinks into the shadow realm. From there, it can, as we now know, make its presence felt in a variety of ways. Those who see through the meaning of an illness pattern and accept it can bring the "embodied" shadow that was banished from conscious awareness into the shadow domain back into consciousness. This new integration of the aspect that was previously blended out heals us and thereby makes us whole. It is an act of shadow integration. Every time we bring a repressed or rejected pole back into conscious awareness, this unification of opposing poles brings us closer to unity. If the asthmatic learns to let go and give freely when breathing out, the asthma condition will be healed. Nevertheless, this situation shows how difficult it is, once a pole of reality has been excluded, to bring it back into consciousness.

It cannot be repeated often enough: as soon as we banish something from consciousness because it scares us, it becomes unconscious and sinks into the shadow domain. Wherever we remove the light of consciousness, we create shadow. However, what has been banished does not give up without a fight. The American psychologist and shadow expert Debbie Ford explains this as follows: "The feelings that we have suppressed are desperate to be integrated into ourselves. They are only harmful when they are repressed: then they can pop up at the least opportune times. Their sneak attacks will handicap you in the areas of your life that mean the most."[5]

In contrast, in the future, we will no longer need to waste huge amounts of effort repressing or fearing any of the characteristics or forms of energy that we become aware of. Quite the contrary,

---

5 Debbie Ford: *The Dark Side of the Light Chasers*. Hodder & Stoughton: London, 2001, pgs 2f.

we can make good use of them instead of letting them abuse and torture us. If we do not deal voluntarily with the shadow, it will deal with us in its own way. This is not intended as a threat, but is instead simply a certainty and ray of hope at the same time.

Throughout the ages people have known, or at least suspected what the underlying pattern of the human development path is: it is modelled on the course of the sun, our central celestial body. Seen from the Earth, the sun also appears to wander through the shadow realm. This is the primordial pattern of polarity.

In this world of opposites, we are all like the Babylonian sun hero Gilgamesh. Gilgamesh had to wrestle with his dark twin Enkidu in order to overcome the challenges of his life path and win over his shadow as his most important ally. We all have to learn to deal with the polarity of this world, which is dominated by contrasts, in order to come closer to God, respectively to unity. Abel had to clash with Cain. Adam finds his opposite pole in Eva, the Hindu God Shiva in his wife Parvati.

It is only for fans of positive thinking with their affirmation acrobatics and sporting stars who rely on doping for their victories that a direct flight into the light seems like a realistic dream. Those who achieve success using methods such as these that are regarded as cheating will never truly be able to enjoy their triumph. In contrast, those who have managed to overcome the deep gorge that lay before the climb to the top, thereby mastering the lows before the highs, will celebrate their success in a different way, namely as a unified whole. They have come to know both sides of their (life) path. In fairy tales, the hero must assertively set off into the unknown in order to learn the meaning of real fear. Only then can he step up as the rightful heir to the throne and claim the hand of the princess. It is the journey into the darkness of his soul that makes him strong enough.

Athletes know that every training session at first weakens them, so that they at first experience a drop in performance before they then regenerate and reach a higher level. They thus work their way upwards in a gradually increasing wave pattern, which represents the typical course of development in an archetypal sense.

The experience with shadow is an integral part of the human development path. We have to learn to love our enemy, before we can become one with him. Anyone interested in self-development will run up against this fact and necessarily also up against shadow. Only the words for it vary. Buddha taught that before our final release, we have to become conscious of all earlier incarnations, both those as the victim and those as the perpetrator. Elizabeth Kübler-Ross, a researcher who specialized in death and dying, strongly encouraged people to take care of unfinished business, so that they could end their lives harmoniously. The therapist Bert Hellinger notes that every system strives for completeness. To put it simply, we have to clean up the past before we can arrive healthy and whole in the present. That is also the essential goal of reincarnation/shadow therapy, which uses previous incarnations to let go of old ballast and burdens and to become free to enjoy the here and now.

The light of awakenment, of enlightenment, needs shadow as urgently as breathing in needs breathing out. To put it another way, the human path of development leads through polarity, the world of contrasts. Both poles of reality are equally important and cannot do without each other. The destination at the end of this path is the overcoming of polarity, by achieving unity. All religions are in agreement in this respect. At first glance, the law of polarity seems to be so simple, so obvious, that dealing with it does not seem to be worth the effort. A closer look, however, reveals that there is more to polarity than meets the eye. Shadow is a child of polarity—typically the most important, but at the same time, usually the most neglected one. We will approach this topic as simply as possible in order to be able to use it to develop ourselves and achieve freedom.

In our polar world, everything exists *natur(e)*ally in terms of contrasts: no-one could feel tall, if there weren't others who were small(er). Peace is not imaginable without war, rich without poor and even good without evil. From our perspective, living in a world of opposites, we cannot even imagine unity. Polarity forces us to perceive everything in terms of contrast. From the perspective of unity, everything is naturally one. In line with this, the contrasts belong together and are only complete when they are together. That we continually overlook this fact is the major mistake that we make in our polar world.

Practical Exercise

Try to think of something in this world that does not have an opposite pole. After you have experienced the futility of this experience, spend a moment enjoying the certainty that necessarily follows from this that you also have a dark side.

Record any thoughts you have about this in your shadow diary.

The creation of our world

Polarity develops from unity. This already becomes clear from the very first verse of the Bible: "In the beginning, God created Heaven and Earth". God stands for unity, Heaven and Earth stand for the world of opposites. After this first step into polarity, it continues accordingly: God creates light and separates it from darkness, then separates the land from the water and so on. Accordingly, the first ten verses of *Genesis* deal with the division of what was previously one into pairs of opposites. The idea that the world developed from the division of unity into opposites forms the basis of almost all religions. In Chinese, for example, the unity of Tao becomes the polarity of Yin, the dark, moist Earth element, and Yang, the bright, fixed Heaven element. The *Tao Te Ching* describes this division of unity in the second verse:

> When people see some things as beautiful,
> other things become ugly.
> When people see some things as good,
> other things become bad.
>
> Being and non-being create each other.
> Difficult and easy support each other.
> Long and short define each other.
> High and low depend on each other.
> Before and after follow each other.
>
> Therefore the Master acts
> without doing anything
> and teaches without saying anything.
> Things arise and she lets them come;
> things disappear and she lets them go.
> She has but doesn't possess,
> acts but doesn't expect.
> When her work is done, she forgets it.
> That is why it lasts forever.[6]

Similarly, the Bible describes the world of opposites by bringing the concept of time into play, which is foreign to unity:

> There is a time for everything,
> and a season for every activity under the heavens:
> a time to be born
> and a time to die,

6 Laozi, & Stephen Mitchell. *Tao Te Ching: A New English Version*. New York: Harper & Row, 1988. Print.

a time to plant
and a time to uproot,
a time to kill
and a time to heal,
a time to tear down
and a time to build,
a time to weep
and a time to laugh,
a time to mourn
and a time to dance,
a time to scatter stones
and a time to gather them,
a time to embrace
and a time to refrain from embracing,
a time to search
and a time to give up,
a time to keep
and a time to throw away,
a time to tear
and a time to mend,
a time to be silent
and a time to speak,
a time to love
and a time to hate,
a time for war
and a time for peace.[7]

Geometry provides an illustration of our worldly problem with unity—a concept, which we are not able to imagine, given that our sensory organs also obey polarity and are based on comparison. A (one-dimensional) point can probably be thought of at least theoretically, but not perceived physically. For this, it would need some form of extension, and a (two-dimensional) disk would result, if not a (three-dimensional) sphere.

7 *Holy Bible, New International Version®, NIV®* Copyright © 1973, 1978, 1984, 2011 by Biblica, Inc.®. All rights reserved worldwide.

Meditation

Read Meditations 1 & 2 aloud to yourself.

Allow yourself sufficient time for the impact of the meditation to sink in and to come to a harmonious close.

Finally, return to the here and now with a deep breath that re-connects you with polarity and the world of contrasts. Re-orient yourself consciously in space by slowly stretching and moving your body, and in time, by taking a look at your watch.

Record your impressions in your shadow diary.

Allowing in light and consciousness

In the end, there is only unity, but in our world, it remains invisible to the human eye. In keeping with the concept of ultimate reality, however, unity stands far above the polarity that permeates it at every level and at every moment. It is only in a world of polarity that the shadow appears equal to the light, with light itself also being a symbol of unity. When it comes to ultimate reality, in contrast, light stands above shadow. Whereas the shadow represents the absence of consciousness, and as such, is nothing on its own and lacks independence, the light (of consciousness) exists in and of itself and does not need the shadow to do so.

A familiar example makes this clear: A tiny candle is enough to drive away the darkness. But if we consider things the other way round, the shadow cannot affect the light. The relationship of light and shadow in the world can further be illustrated by the image of a developmental triangle that is shown below: its upper tip stands as a symbol for unity (1), the base below for polarity with its two poles (2) and (3). If we divide the triangle from the tip down into two halves, the darkest black as a symbol of shadow and bright light stand opposite each other at the base of the triangle. With each developmental step that we achieve in the course of our life, and thus each higher level in the triangle, the light on the bright side remains equally bright, but on the shadow side, the blackness decreases. As consciousness grows, the absence of light diminishes, and the shadow is ultimately illuminated more and more, transforming first to dark grey then to light grey. Near the top, it becomes particularly clear that, whereas the light does not change, the shadow gradually disappears or simply dissolves into the light.

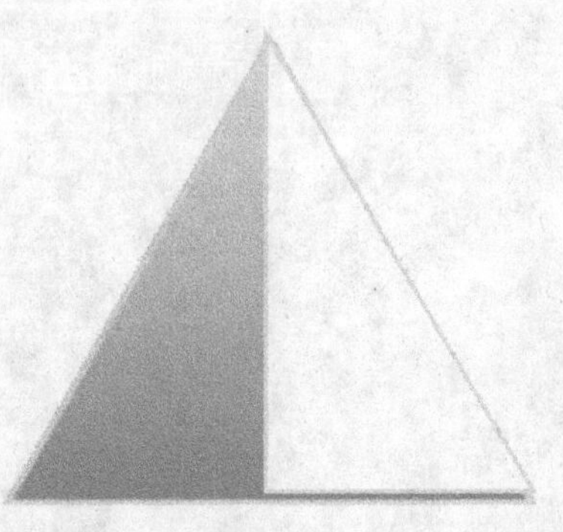

This means that the greatest brightness and the darkest shadows clash most strongly at the base of the triangle. The light on this lower level corresponds to the conscious Self or Ego; at this level of development, the Ego is necessary for our survival.

On the path to the pinnacle of the triangle, the Self needs the contrast of the shadow as its opposite to become more and more conscious.

During this process, the shadow becomes weaker or more transparent; and correspondingly, in our triangle image, greyer and finally lighter. The higher we rise in our development, the brighter the shadow becomes, or in other words, the more the light penetrates into its territory. This process can also be called healing.

At the highest point of the triangle, both sides pass into the light of oneness, which corresponds to the divine light and the Self. The light no longer has a counterpart and is beyond the polar world, or in other words, is everywhere at the same time. Only now are we truly in reality and can finally realize that the path to this point and the world of polarity—with its light and shadow, including all of its difficulties and deceptions—were nothing more than illusion. This or something similar is how people who have found fulfilment describe this experience. In the *Tao Te Ching* this is expressed in verse 41 as follows:

> The path into the light seems dark,
> the path forward seems to go back,
> the direct path seems long,
> true power seems weak,
> true purity seems tarnished,
> true steadfastness seems changeable,
> true clarity seems obscure,
> the greatest care seems unsophisticated,
> the greatest love seems indifferent,
> the greatest wisdom seems childish.
>
> The Tao is nowhere to be found.
> Yet it nourishes and completes all things[8]

Self-actualization involves illuminating the shadow and making it conscious. It equates to the dissolution of ego and shadow as both merge into the Self. In actual fact, however, they do not truly disappear, but instead become the energy source of the Self in a transformed form. In a similar way, Enkidu does not disappear in the myth, but instead develops into Gilgamesh's source of strength. In the figurative expression of "being one with everything", the Self corresponds to the experience of non-differentiation. What is represented schematically in the image of the development triangle is expressed more vividly in the *Tao Te Ching*. Unity does not only exist at the top of the triangle, of course, but instead is always everywhere; we simply do not see

8 Ibid Laotse & Stephen Mitchell

it and we continually try to understand it in terms of our polar imagery. The Lebanese poet Khalil Gibran beautifully describes the battle between light and shadow in his story *Satan*. Satan, wounded in battle by the Archangel Michael, asks a priest to save him:

"I am the enraged and mute tempest who agitates the minds of man and the hearts of women. And in fear of me, they will travel to places of worship to condemn me, or to places of vice to make me happy by surrendering to my will. The monk who prays in the silence of the night to keep me away from his bed is like the prostitute who invites me to her chamber. I am Satan everlasting and eternal.

I am the builder of convents and monasteries upon the foundation of fear. I build wine shops and wicked houses upon the foundations of lust and self-gratification. If I cease to exist, fear and enjoyment will be abolished from the world, and through their disappearance, desires and hopes will cease to exist in the human heart. Life will become empty and cold, like a harp with broken strings. I am Satan everlasting.

I am the inspiration of falsehood, slander, treachery, deceit and mockery, and if these elements were to be removed from this world, human society would become like a deserted field in which naught would thrive but thorns of virtue. I am Satan everlasting.

I am the father and mother of sin, and if sin were to vanish, the fighters of sin would vanish with it, along with their families and structures."

The priest replies:

"I know now what I had not known an hour ago. Forgive my ignorance. I know that your existence in this world creates temptation, and temptation is a measurement by which God adjudges the value of human souls. It is a scale which Almighty God uses to weigh the spirits. I am certain that if you die, temptation will die, and with its passing, death will destroy the ideal power which elevates and alerts man.

You must live, for if you die and the people know it, their fear of hell will vanish and they will cease worshipping, for naught would be sin. You must live, for in your life is the salvation of humanity from vice and sin.

As to myself, I shall sacrifice my hatred for you on the altar of my love for man."[9]

This theme is expressed in a more modern form in the film *The Devil's Advocate*. In it, Al Pacino plays an enchantingly

9 www.newthoughtlibrary.com *Satan* by Khalil Gibran

Film Meditation

Watch the film *The Devil's Advocate* with a meditative attitude. Recognize and value it as an excursion into the shadow realm in all its facets. Be consciously aware right from the start that all of its characters are a part of you and will therefore have affected you in some way or other (this applies also for all of the remaining film meditations in this book). Whenever you notice that you are identifying with one of the main actors—for example, the hero, played by Keanu Reeves, or with the beautiful victim played by Charlize Theron, remain conscious at the same time, that both characters exist within you, and that above and beyond these, all of the other characters exists within you, too, even the grand seducer portrayed by Al Pacino.

Directly after this "film meditation", as soon as the magic words "The End" appear on the DVD, the actual exercise should begin (this also applies for further film meditations. Close your eyes to the external world and turn your attention within, asking yourself what this film about shadow has to do with you, what it evokes within in you and what it tells you about yourself.

Make appropriate notes in your shadow diary.

seductive devil, whose charm neither the man of principle nor the religious zealot can resist.

Self-actualization

Seen from our level of existence, everything appears in opposites. In fact, this is the only way that we can even perceive anything at all. As a result, opposites, and with them polarity itself, are the only possibility we have for getting closer to unity—perfection or the divine. Since shadow is the ultimate result of polarity formation, illumination of the shadow can also best bring us (back) to unity. Whatever form the shadow may take, it represents our greatest chance, and we should learn to see through its disguise and recognize it as an opportunity. In other words, it is from the darkness of our unconsciousness that our self-actualization or liberation is born. We must ascend from darkness to light, just as Creation materialized from light. This symbolism is celebrated with the ritual of the winter solstice. It is at the time of the shortest day, when the light is weakest and the darkness is deepest that, symbolically, (the son of) God, the light of the world, is born. The same is expressed in the lotus flower, the Buddhist and Hindu symbol for the highest level of purity. In this respect, it is said that it is from the deepest dirt, i.e. the mud of the pond, that the thousand-petaled lotus—as the symbol of enlightenment—blooms.

The fact that we reach the light by passing through the darkness, or in other words, that we achieve liberation through integrating the shadow was expressed by C.G. Jung in the formula: Ego + Shadow = Self. The Ego is everything that we consciously identify with. It includes all of the well-accepted qualities that others attribute to us, respectively all of the abilities that we are consciously aware of. Shadow, on the other hand, is everything that is unconscious for us. Consequently, it contains everything that we have rejected, everything negative that others have attributed to us, and all of the criticism and abuse that we refuse to accept and have thus banished from consciousness. In order to reach our Self, which represents the highest stage in our development towards liberation, and consequently, self-actualization, the Ego and the Shadow, or our bright conscious and dark unconscious side must come together. This is the goal of shadow, respectively, reincarnation therapy. Whenever psychotherapy chooses self-actualization and liberation as its goal, the shadow must therefore become its primary task.

Anyone who understands the Law of Polarity in the sense of my book *The Laws of Fate* knows how closely both poles are connected and how easily we often reach the desired pole via its opposite pole. For example, javelin throwers and shot-putters lean far in the other direction before they hurl their weapons towards the target. Gardeners who water exquisite roses with foul-smelling liquid manure instead of sweet perfume are also following this wisdom. Religions and the spiritual wisdom of old teach us that the freedom that modern people yearn for so deeply can only be achieved through voluntary submission to this law. The *Tao Te Ching* expresses this in verse 22 as follows:

> If you want to become whole,
> let yourself be partial.
> If you want to become straight,
> let yourself be crooked.
> If you want to become full,
> let yourself be empty.
> If you want to be reborn,
> let yourself die.
> If you want to be given everything,
> give everything up.[10]

Paradoxes of the sort that are frequently used in the *Tao Te Ching* are still the best way to shed light on unity from our plane of polarity. Nevertheless, most people insist on following the direct path of sticking to just one pole, and even repeated failure

10 Ibid Laotse & Stephen Mitchell

is not enough to sway them from their course. Driven to despair, they continue to seek success in a one-sided way, without ever taking the opposite pole or shadow into consideration. The lack of success stories along this (wrong) track also rarely manages to set them straight. In contrast, the life stories of self-actualized people and saints show how much they relied on both poles.

Shadow diary

Am I already miles away from my actual destination and right in the middle of the opposite pole? Have I sometimes only noticed in retrospect just how much shadow I ended up mobilizing with my actions? With this dilemma in mind, can I relate to Berthold Brecht's realization that "the opposite of good is not evil, it is good intention".

Write down your thoughts on this.

How shadow is built up

Our learning of the basic instructions for shadow production begins early in life. "Make up your mind!", "Either or!"—these are the maxims that surround us from our earliest childhood onward, and every decision inevitably leads to the creation of shadow. The choice of one direction necessarily excludes at least one other direction. A "both-this-and-that" approach would actually be a more appropriate fit for reality, because it would leave room for both poles. Our society, however, is more focused on making decisions and combating opposites than on integrating both sides and cooperating. In this respect, we have a lot to learn if we are to be able to deal with the great shadow issues facing our society and our world. Every fixed state ultimately amounts to remaining stuck in a single pole, and as such, promotes the creation of shadow. Reality is more accurately described by Heraclitus's "*Panta rhei*" ("Everything flows"). Despite this, fixed states, strong positions and firm, immovable standpoints continue to be extremely popular. Ideally, politicians are supposed to never change their minds. To ensure that this does not happen after all, their opinions are kept in check by so-called "factional pressure". To toe the line with this compulsive force, these elected representatives of the people are not supposed to follow their conscience or what they feel to be their mission. Instead, they are expected to support the power aspirations of their party leaders.

When Christ calls the Devil the "Lord of this world", he recognizes him as the "King of polarity". This is symbolized in the duality of his horns. When we, as children in this world of contrasts, are constantly forced to choose between these poles or opposites—preferring one and excluding the other—we are constantly producing shadow, and as a result, are helping the "Lord of the shadow kingdom" to do his work. Conversely, the latter is always helping the good side to do its work at the same time. The famous sentence from Goethe's Faust makes this clear: the devil (Mephisto) is actually always trying to create evil, but ends up, however reluctantly, always creating good. In psychotherapy, too, the shadow or the unconscious, is our most valuable helper.

One of the more major problems of our world is that so many people who think they are good do not notice at all how much they are actually helping the forces of evil to do their work; for example, when George W. Bush, with his "war on terror", in actual fact, is the person who most strongly fans the flames. Or when Edward Jenner, the inventor of vaccination, realizes on his deathbed that, instead of endowing mankind with a blessing, he has actually created a monster. The medical study, which uncovered that every antibiotic treatment administered in the first two years of life increases the risk of a person later becoming an allergy sufferer by more than fifty percent, also reveals shadow.

Handling evil

Before anyone is too quick to reach the inverse conclusion that all they need to do is to commit evil in order to achieve good, a clear warning upfront is in order. All of this is far more about recognizing and owning up to evil in ourselves and our (his)story in order to achieve greater consciousness. If someone were to commit evil deeds on purpose, they would simply give birth to new shadow in the world, which they—as is the case with everything that originates from them—would once again have to answer for. In relation to this, there is a story by Jean Tinder about the light and the dark within all of us: One evening, an old Cherokee Indian was telling his grandson a story about the battle that rages within all people. "My boy!" he said, "This battle rages within each and every one of us like a fight between two wolves. One of them represents evil. He is anger, envy, jealousy, conceitedness, suffering, hatred, greed, arrogance, self-pity, dislike, inferiority, lies, pride, desire, superiority and egoism. The other represents good. He is joy, peace, love, hope, composure, humanity, kindness, goodness, empathy, generosity, truth, compassion and trust." The grandson thought about it for a while and then asked: "Grandfather, which wolf wins?" The old Cherokee replied, "The one you feed."

What this means is that we are, of course, welcome to keep doing good. Nevertheless, at the same time, it makes

Shadow diary

In which situation might I enjoy consciously doing something evil, living out shadow? What could tempt me to go to extremes? Have there been outbreaks of shadow in my life so far, for example, in the form of unconscious aggression or meanness.

Record anything that occurs to you in this regard in your diary.

sense to also be watchful and open to the shadow that is constantly developing. This is the reason why the Native American cultures had the Heyoka—a kind of holy fool. Whenever something was decided on, this person played the naysayer, and as part of a ritual, demanded the opposite of what had just been decided. In this way, the Heyoka made the downside or shadow side visible. The court jesters of the Middle Ages played a similar role.

Shadow is, to put it simply, everything that we do not want to see in ourselves and in our world. Since we spend our whole lives yearning for some things and rejecting others, our shadow grows with us. The older we get, the larger and more powerful it becomes—at least to the extent that we do not become aware of it and do not choose to actively confront it. Of course, the longer our journey through life lasts, the more difficult this becomes. But, precisely because shadow represents the collection of all those things and characteristics that we have not accepted in ourselves and in our world throughout our lives, they remain attached to us—albeit unconsciously and in shadow form. Nevertheless, a positive aspect, such as courage, can also be part of the shadow if it has been overlooked by cowardly people as a possibility. Naturally, the part of the shadow that causes us the most trouble and that has been granted the largest amount of space in this book is the part that is regarded as evil.

While we ourselves cannot see our shadow, others are more than able to do so. That is why older people who are not aware of polarity seem so embarrassing to those around them. Their own image of themselves matches less and less with the perception of others. As people get older and older, this discrepancy also shows up more and more clearly in their behaviour as well, and others are thus able to see through it even more quickly. For example, those who are constantly emphasizing their own honesty soon raise suspicions amongst others regarding dishonesty. The *Tao Te Ching*'s solution to dealing with "evil" is neither aimed at fighting against "evil" deeds, nor aimed at any pole at all. In this respect, verse 60 states:

Governing a large country
is like frying a small fish.
You spoil it with too much poking.

Center your country in the Tao
and evil will have no power.
Not that it isn't there,
but you'll be able to step out of its way.

Give evil nothing to oppose
and it will disappear by itself.[11]

---

11 Ibid Laotse & Stephen Mitchell

Resistance to Reality or Acceptance

Finding a reliable basis

Basically, we can accept reality as it is or fight against it. The latter leads, for example, to war. If we want to change reality, we can first accept it as it is and then try to actively reshape it, for instance, by means of political action—or to transform it by changing ourselves. The latter represents a highly underestimated, but wonderful opportunity. Trying to effect change by making demands on our environment seems to be the easier way and is therefore the preferred option for most people. The results, however, are depressing. Typically, the only thing that whiners, bellyachers and complainers achieve is that they can barely bear themselves anymore. The path recommended in this book is to first accept reality as you find it and to change yourself rather than demanding or trying to force change through in the external world. This path is very successful, but at the same time, very demanding and for many very unfamiliar.Rhythm arises from the constant alternation between two poles and is essential for life. Rudolf Steiner, the founder of anthroposophy, was of the opinion that all life itself is nothing but rhythm. It is certainly true that life unfolds in the world

Putting our own house in order first tends to be an unpopular option for us, even though it is a very effective one. Most people have instead shifted their focus to projection, or passing the buck, thus turning this into a kind of mass sport that enjoys widespread popularity. At first glance, nothing seems easier than denying all responsibility and laying the blame on someone else's doorstep. On top of this, constant self-defence strategies and the tactic of counterattacking (in keeping with the motto "you're no better yourself") leave the shadow untouched and get in the way of further development.

Most of our problems stem from various forms of resistance, and consequently, the constant battle or even the full-scale war against reality, and as a result of this, also against the truth. The key question is whether this war is really worth it. Is it not simply a whole lot better to just live with the truth within reality?

Many of our problems quickly turn into a constant stream of reproaches: our partner should not be having an affair; we should be earning more money; our kids should help around the house more; the rich and powerful should be more considerate, politicians more honest and caring, our taxes lower, our in-laws more respectful, cleaning ladies more efficient, doctors more committed, bosses more generous, tradespeople more competent, psychotherapists more empathetic; and the symptoms of any illness I have should also have cleared up long ago.

The basis for our reproaches is dissatisfaction, more precisely a kind of rebellion against Creation. This quickly becomes evident with the reciting of the Lord's Prayer "Thy Will be done on earth as it is in heaven" is the actual instruction. Instead, however, modern humans, to the extent that they even still pray at all, think "Dear God, I have a few wishes, please arrange things accordingly ..." It thus all boils down to the exact opposite, namely "My will be done". If this will is not able to push its way through, a new sense of dissatisfaction and further reproaches develop.

The Germans are well-known worldwide, if not to say downright notorious, for criticizing so many things and constantly wanting to improve them. Nevertheless, this is the general attitude in modern society. We are chronically dissatisfied, are continually finding fault with reality and believe that it should kindly adjust to our expectations as quickly as possible. We do not just place orders for the Cosmos to fulfil, we actively direct complaints towards it. With both forms of expression, we are stating that God should arrange things better (for us). In contrast, how much wiser is the eastern realization "What you want will happen or something better" or even the good old "Thy Will be done". The modern attitude, which makes happiness dependent on getting everything you want, unfortunately leads us in a goal-driven way down a wrong track via dissatisfaction straight into unhappiness. In contrast, we reach happiness when we want everything we get.

Since, in the end, reality does not adjust itself to our expectations in response to complaints or orders or wishlists, many of us are in a constant state of stress and loaded with reproaches and improvement suggestions. Seeing through this modern attitude and re-evaluating it is helpful and important.

Shadow diary

Part one: What are my personal demands and improvement suggestions? What could I do to realize these myself? What do I believe I deserve instead? How should my life look? How should the world function for me to be in agreement with it? What could God or Creation learn from me and do better in the future?

Please list everything.

In terms of our own self-development, experience shows just how ineffective years of kicking up a storm against reality and directing never-ending accusations and complaints to the highest authority actually ends up being. Instead, these aspects merely lead to screwed-up lives full of anger directed towards an army of alleged culprits. Those who spend years complaining that their partner, their boss, their money situation should be different, overlook the simple reality that these things are, in fact, not different. There is only one sensible way out of this situation: namely, acknowledging reality as it truly is as quickly as possible. It is never too late to do this. Reality is also never offended. It simply keeps on operating in the same way and does not care at all about the whiners and bellyachers.

The sooner we give up our resistance to reality, the better it is for ourselves. There is no intelligent alternative to acknowledging what actually is. Only then does it make sense to begin deciding whether we should try to change the external reality that we have finally acknowledged, for example, through political action or different rituals, or whether we should turn our attention inwards and change ourselves instead.

Shadow diary

Part two: How much substance is there to my personal reproaches? Are they actually true and realistic? And what do they do for me? And those around me? Is there any chance of changing the reality that is being criticized by means of such reproaches? Or should I perhaps instead change the reproaches, and accept myself, and in doing so, also accept reality. Which of my reproaches could I already give up on in these sense of "Thy Will be done".

Confide the results of this talk with yourself to your shadow

In order to acknowledge what is, we do not have to find it beautiful or appreciate and praise it. Acceptance simply means no longer whining and complaining about what we have been given and ceasing to kick up a storm against it (internally or externally). Those who complain that their partner has been cheating on them for years, do not want to change anything. They just want to whine and lay blame. Their energy flows into the whining, and this represents a highly questionable way of wasting energy, as this is then lacking for dealing with the situation.

In accordance with the Law of Resonance, even listening to people who continually complain is already highly questionable. Those who spend a lot of time with gossipers are known to become gossipers themselves. The same happens to those who spend a lot of time with whiners.

We should also take the words of Marcus Aurelius very seriously, who said: "Over time, the soul takes on the colour of your thoughts". In this way, many people become the creators of precisely the reality they wish to avoid. We shape our own reality through our belief system.

Acknowledging and accepting reality as it is offers the best chance of long-term success in life. On top of that, it is an amazing source of power. Religious people who feel accepted by God just the way they are are usually well ahead of others. To give a relevant example: When mental training first emerged and was being intensively used in sports, there were some very successful top skiers of the ski elite who chose to do without additional help of this type. When questioned, it turned out that they always felt accepted, loved and supported by God or their partner, regardless of whether they won or lost. On this basis, nothing could actually happen to them. This in turn produced exactly the sense of safety that was needed to win more often than average—with below-average numbers of falls and injuries. The careers of stars like the Swiss Pirmin Zurbriggen, the German Markus Wasmeier or the Austrian Petra Kronberger are good examples of this.

As long as people continue to deny reality and persuade themselves, for example, that they only drink a few too many now and then, they will never be able to overcome their alcoholism. This can only succeed if they admit to it. This is also the central basis for the success of Alcoholics Anonymous. Those affected fully acknowledge their dilemma. Only then can they get down to brass tacks and count on the support of Fate. As long as I continue to lie to myself, I have no energy for the upcoming fight for my life. The *Tao Te Ching* formulates this connection in the 71st verse as follows:

> First realize that you are sick;
> then you can move toward health.
> The Master is her own physician.[12]

Those who complain about external or internal circumstances simply end up keeping these alive by doing so. What is more, they become the creator of their own vale of tears. Whiners do not want to change anything, and in fact never do, even if they profess the opposite. If you confront them with this head-on, they get angry, which serves to confirm the suspicion.

A further illustrative example: In my many years as a fasting doctor and medical expert on nutrition, I have yet to experience that anyone who made excuses based on hormones, their glands, a weak metabolism or their inherited predisposition actually managed to get their obesity under control. In contrast, after honestly admitting to their eating problem, many others did manage to solve it and reach their ideal figure. Along the way, knowledge of hormones and glands can, of course, be helpful.

Similarly, among those around me, nobody has ever managed to solve their personal financial problems while projecting these onto "our unjust economic system". Those projecting in this way all remained obsessed with money and their personal problems with it. Nevertheless, many others have managed to get it under control by taking personal responsibility for it in the sense of my book *The Psychology of Money**. In doing so, they started possessing their money instead of being possessed by it. It is not so difficult to gain freedom at this level if the basic facts are accepted.

Reality keeps on working whether we choose to acknowledge it or not. For this reason, we might as well just do so. There is simply no other alternative. Only if we are able to accept the

---

12 Ibid Laotse & Stephen Mitchell

external reality that we find around us can we succeed in it. And only if we are able to accept our own inner reality can we successfully develop ourselves and become the creators of our own reality. Nevertheless, this has to be preceded by the humble acceptance of the place that Creation has assigned to us for the time being. Gitta Mallasz formulates this in the following way: "If you bow your head and feel uplifted—this is true humility.

If you bow your head and feel lowered—this is false humility.[13]

As therapists, we have to meet our patients where they are currently at and not where we would like them to be. Similarly, if I am a person seeking to develop myself further, I also have to meet myself where I currently am and not where I would like to be. Acceptance of what is is therefore the only reliable basis for development and shadow work.

If we want to develop in the outside world, for example in a financial sense, we also must be prepared to accept the conditions that we find in the outside world if we wish to be able to influence them in our favour. If I want to develop spiritually, I have to accept myself the way I am now in order to continue from here in the direction that I have in mind.

Nevertheless, it is important to recognise clearly that accepting something does not necessarily mean approving of or even supporting it. It may not even mean tolerating something over a longer period. It simply means giving up our resistance right now, in this moment, in the present, and accepting something in our own reality exactly the way it is now. The alcoholic must therefore accept his or her alcoholism right now in this moment and by no means continue to tolerate it a single day more.

Acceptance means giving up the denial of reality and instead taking note of whatever our current reality is and considering it noteworthy, no matter how it has turned out. Only those who are able to view things in this way will learn the truth and be operating within reality. From this point onwards, they can immediately start working on themselves and their patterns. Or as the

---

13 Gitta Mallasz: *Talking with Angels*. Daimon, Einsiedeln, 1988, pg 84.

Buddhist Thich Nhat Hanh suggests: "Embrace your unaccepted patterns of behavior, your dark sides in the loving way that a mother does with a crying a child—in that moment, you begin to transform them."[14]

Anyone who acknowledges the reality that they are in and makes honest decisions starting from this level is free to be bold and daring and to undertake demanding and even tremendous feats. In doing so, they will receive the support of destiny and experience the immense energies that flow from reality and truth. These energies affect all levels—from sufficient neurotransmitters to the right social relationships and the acquisition of the necessary skills. Those who make honest and binding decisions, for example, in the sense of the formerly more widespread word of honour can rely not only on themselves, but also on Fate. Their word is granted magical power and their role in life given more meaning. The 28th verse of the *Tao Te Ching* says:[15]

> "Accept the world as it is.
> If you accept the world,
> the Tao will be luminous inside you
> and you will return to your primal self."

---

14 Thich Nhat Hanh: *Heute achtsam leben.* 366 inspirierende Gedanken. Herder, Freiburg 1999

15 Ibid Laotse & Stephen Mitchell

Meditation

Read meditation 1 and 3 aloud to yourself and allow yourself sufficient time afterwards for the meditation to come to a harmonious close.

Return to the here and now by taking a deep breath. Re-orient yourself consciously in space by stretching and moving your body, and in time, by taking a look at your watch.

Record your impressions in your shadow diary

Projection traps

We are all too happy to look for the causes of our problems in the outside world, even though, in reality, the causes lie within ourselves, and instead, we shift the blame for this onto others by means of projection. Nevertheless, this behavior does not provide us with a solution. The *Tao Te Ching* draws our attention to this particular danger, which we are very fond of ignoring: "If you shift the blame onto someone else, there is no end to the accusations.[16]

Despite this, many people in today's world believe more strongly than ever in the issuing of blame to others. Everything unpleasant is projected as far away as possible onto others, who know nothing about it and who are thus unable to consciously defend themselves against it. The method is extremely easy to see through, but nonetheless still continues to find many supporters, as the following joke illustrates: When a doctor asks a man about the cause of the severe burns on his ears, he answers: "I was ironing when the phone rang. I accidentally put the iron to my ear instead of the phone." The doctor is astounded, "But why is your other ear so burnt?" he asks. The patient answers, "Because the idiot called again!"

16 Ibid Laotse & Stephen Mitchell

What defence is there then against the projections of others? Since manifestations can only occur through resonance, this also represents the only sensible way to defend ourselves. If we protest too much and try to shield ourselves against the accusations, we all too easily become a person with precisely the qualities concerned. To put it another way, if you label someone as being in a bad mood for long enough, that will actually eventually be enough to put them in a bad mood after all. Even if they still vigorously defend themselves by denying the projection at the beginning, in the end, they will react with bad-temperedness and thus eventually prove the person doing the projecting right. It is important to see through this tricky mechanism and to focus on avoiding the corresponding resonance.[17] On the other hand, those who do not build up any resonance with a particular topic will not attract any projections in this respect either.

Something as evident as the Law of Resonance has long been ignored and is only now receiving long overdue recognition. In the past, instead of dealing with the subject of resonance, various sciences, such as sociology and psychology emerged, which were partly dedicated to the debt projection game: The external circumstances, our socialisation, our parents, and more recently, the environment are supposedly to blame for everything. By digging in its heels over a long period of time, Freudian psychoanalysis has sat it out long enough to acquire a kind of recognition status that puts it in the position to project a lot of blame or responsibility onto parents, and especially mothers, at the expense of the health insurance companies. The question is what, besides relieving our own conscience, is this actually supposed to achieve? Has such a scientifically-disguised system of debt projection ever permanently healed any kind of symptom?

The age-old wisdom that, for the most part, the problem always lies with the one pointing the finger at others, is revealed with beautiful clarity in the gesture itself. As is well known, only

---

17 More on this in the chapters about resonance in *Die Schicksalsgesetze* (*The Laws of Fate**); Book list available at www.dahlke.at/buecherliste and the CD *Gesetz der Anziehung* (The Law of Attraction CD*)

two fingers point towards the accused, while three point back to the person who is actually responsible, namely the owner of the hand.

There is little that can be changed in the outside world. Who would ever dream of trying to successfully squeeze out a pimple in the mirror itself? Naturally, we can only ever see it clearly in the mirror, which makes the mirror itself extremely necessary. In a case like this, however, we are aware of the projection and that the pimple is not really there in the mirror. Nevertheless, as soon as our morning visit to the bathroom is behind us, the same impressive game of projection begins worldwide. In the process, the majority of social workers and politicians all try to remedy the state of human misery in the outside world. This is certainly well-intentioned, but of course, their actual level of success leaves a lot to be desired.

In practice though, the debt projection game is not limited to politicians and the aforementioned sciences; it can, in fact, be found everywhere: from business to education, and in all kinds of personal domains. In this respect, it has also become a very common game between partners, and probably has as many relationships on its conscience as the theme of jealousy.

Meditation

Read meditation 1 and 4 aloud to yourself and allow yourself sufficient time afterwards for the meditation to come to a harmonious close.

Return to the here and now by taking a deep breath. Re-orient yourself consciously in space by stretching and moving your body, and in time, by taking a look at your watch.

Record your impressions in your shadow diary

Every projection and accusation is a kind of modern-day throwing down of the gauntlet. Nevertheless, in this way, we give others more energy and ultimately also power over us. As victims of projection, we can be thrown off balance on this point at any time. Not only does this remind us of our shadow aspects, and with these, also our weak points, but also allows others to seize on these aspects and use them to their own advantage. The main problem with projection, however, is the warped view of the world that follows from it, and with this, also a flood of misunderstandings and confusion. It is this that forms the basis for condemnation and prejudice, discrimination and favouritism, sanctimony and bigotry. When we take back our projections, for example by doing shadow work with the help of this book, we take back our power and energy and thus become stronger ourselves without weakening others further. We automatically stop keeping track in the outside world of what we do not want to see in ourselves. As a result, we get back what we had transferred to the outside world and connect more intensively with our own core essence, our Self. As soon as we free ourselves from the confused entanglement of projections, we see ourselves as we are and the world as it is—and no longer as a mirror of our own (un)desirable characteristics and traits. In this way, the world becomes more beautiful, and we become more real and human, more ourselves.

If the world is merely projection, as conveyed for example in the teachings of Tibetan Buddhism, it can, of course, only be changed within a person. Christ teaches something similar when he speaks of the Kingdom of Heaven lying within us. In fact, this is an assumption that is shared by spiritual philosophy in general. Byron Katie, the American specialist in shadow work, says: "Eventually you come to see that everything outside you is a reflection of your own thinking. You are the storyteller, the projector of all stories, and the world is the projected image of your thoughts"[18]

18 Byron Katie. *Loving What Is: Four Questions that can Change Your Life*. Random House: UK, pg 10

There is much to be said for this world view, as the following anecdote from the world of Greek mythology also demonstrates: following the completion of Creation, Apollo was commissioned with carefully hiding the key to it so that no one would find it. After careful consideration and many suggestions, which even went as far as hiding it on the moon, he had a sudden flash of inspiration. He decided to hide the key inside people, within their hearts, as he knew that that would be the last place they would think to look.

Thus far, history has proven Apollo right. Nowadays, however, we could be finally ready to find the key in our own hearts. More and more people are wising up to their own tricks and are turning inwards on their search. The writer Paolo Coelho presents a variation on this theme in his first and most successful novel *The Alchemist*, which tells the story of how the alchemist embarks on a long journey only to find that the great treasure he is seeking is actually in the home town that he had been in all along and to which he returns in the end. Previously, Janosch had presented a similar story in his world-famous children's book *The Trip to Panama*. The fact that the same general theme has twice managed to produce a world bestseller shows just how (arche)typical it is.

Meditation

Read meditation 1 and 5 aloud to yourself and allow yourself sufficient time afterwards for the meditation to come to a harmonious close.

Return to the here and now by taking a deep breath. Re-orient yourself consciously in space by stretching and moving your body, and in time, by taking a look at your watch.

Record your impressions in your shadow diary

The turnaround game

The fact that, hiding behind the reproaches and accusations that we level against other people, there is always a shadow of our own offers us a wonderful "opportunity", in the truest sense of the word, to deal with these attacks in an extremely effective way. At first glance, the method is very simple. It requires only good will and the willingness to be positively surprised. Ultimately, however, it involves the simple turning around of responsibility in the sense of taking back what we have projected away from us. This automatically takes the load off others, and our life then changes and moves forward in the direction of growth. Doing so also provides us with opportunities for taking action that were previously not at our disposal. Above all, however, it brings the shadow war between people to light, and—if we stick to our responsibility—this shadow war ends up disappearing in the long term with lasting effect.

The main question is simply whether I am willing to "sacrifice" my misery to such a seemingly-simple game. Am I prepared to go along with the following four small tricks (a, b, c and d) in order to transform all the accusations and reproaches that I am currently still nurturing against someone else into growth opportunities for myself and the accused on four different levels?

Although astonishing in its simplicity, the game with pronouns, succeeds in transforming statements that are initially full of reproach and blame into useful clues for our own psychological development. Instead of a statement, such as: "He is deceiving me" (a), three additional levels of observation can be chosen, which directly expose our own shadow, namely: "I am deceiving him" (b), "I am deceiving myself" (c) and "He is deceiving himself" (d).

- Let's take for example a woman and her initial reproach that "he is having an affair and therefore deceiving her" (a).

• This can be turned around and transformed into: "She is deceiving him" (b). This shifts responsibility from him to her, and she becomes capable of acting again.

• Added to this, we also have: "She is deceiving herself" (c), and:

• "He is deceiving himself" (d).

Statements (b) and (c) are more effective in solving the problem than (a) and (d). This is because (b) and (c) are directly in the hands of the woman concerned and thus readily accessible to her, whereas she cannot change anything about (a) and (d). Indirectly, however, she will also be able to gradually influence (a) and (d) via the Law of Resonance.

Without exploring the content any further, any accusation (a) can be turned into its opposite (b) in the sense of such a reversal of blame, or better yet, responsibility. "Peter stole from me" (a) can be transformed to "I stole from Peter" (b). Following this, the other two variants "I stole from myself" (c) and "Peter stole from me" (d) can also be formulated.

As a rule, variants (b), (c) and (d) are more helpful than the original accusation (a). A further concrete and typical example:

"He treats me badly" is the initial accusation made by Lisa towards Franz (a).

"I treat him badly", in other words, Lisa treats Franz badly, represents the turnaround of responsibility (b). If Lisa examines this statement carefully, she will soon hit paydirt as long as she is willing to try looking. If both partners were not actively playing the blame-shifting game, the game would soon come to a standstill and it would not be possible for so much energy to be set in motion. Moreover, in keeping with our shadow theory, any accusation directed at others can always just as easily be directed at oneself. Uncovering the truth is, as the well-known saying goes, "as easy as (a), (b), (c)" (and also (d) in this case!). Once Lisa turns the tables, she will naturally also find incidents in which she has treated Franz badly (b). As she continues to dig deeper, various points that are similar to her own reproaches and that are perhaps even on comparable levels will come to light, not to mention other points and levels of accusation.

Certainly, Franz feels—at least subjectively—that he is also being treated badly by her and that he is not getting what he wants and dreams of getting from her. That he treats her badly (a) is—at least from her point of view—of course, also true. But she cannot directly change that now; she has already tried that long enough. And he has clearly not reacted in a satisfactory way to her reproaches; otherwise, the situation would not have escalated to this point. Obviously, not a nice situation to be in, but undoubtedly Lisa's reality. If she continues to push back against this reality and carries on being reproachful, making demands, seeking allies and just generally projecting, the whole thing will simply escalate further, and in any case, will certainly not improve. Quite the contrary, the fronts will harden instead, and their relationship will slide even further off the rails. Most people take this same track again and again without examining it further—a track which not only bypasses their own shadow, but also all of the opportunities this involves. This applies not only to relationships, but also to all kinds of other issues.

In most cases, Lisa does not have any real chance of changing Franz, even though this is precisely what many women are actually hoping for at the beginning of a relationship and what they have a strong desire to achieve. Despite this, it is practically impossible to reach this goal in this way, and as such, remains an illusion. Insisting on the desired change with ever increasing forcefulness is neither particularly clever nor likely to meet with success. Its only somewhat dubious effect is to enlarge one's own shadow further. Nevertheless, the advantage of this is that those who consider confrontation with their own shadow to be their own responsibility can now see all of these possible accusations and reproaches as an opportunity for their own growth and development. In addition, this simple game, which is, in effect, a form of shadow therapy under one's own direction, will end up improving our relationships with the people around us in a lasting way. This simple change (of sides), Byron Katie speaks of a "turnaround", leads us from the role of victim to perpetrator, from being at the mercy of others to taking responsibility for ourselves, and from being pushed around to becoming a conscious creator.

In our example with Lisa, as soon as she pulls off the easy turnaround (b), she can immediately begin to change something, namely her behavior towards Franz. Instead of treating him badly, she can give him her best, perhaps even offering him more than he expects from her in ways that are even nicer than expected. As a result, he will, in accordance with the Law of Resonance, not only soon stop treating her with contempt, but at some point, will also jump on board the new program of "I give (you) my best ". It is a simply a question of time. Friendliness is well known to act like a boomerang and always comes back eventually. This is not only true for friendliness, however, but for all emotions and feelings, positive as well as negative. The only catch would be that Lisa would have to be nice, even though she appears to be in the right and therefore believes she is entitled to react in an insulted way. It is on this basis that she presumes the necessity, and above all, the right to fight fire with fire. In this respect, she would have to swallow her pride and stop letting these beliefs "overshadow" the relationship in the truest sense of the word.

It is this willingness to take a leap of faith and move beyond our own shadow that is the make-or-break factor for everything. The consequence of refusing to make this leap is that such chains of "reaction and counterreaction" get longer and longer until the relationship breaks apart. Long chains of retaliation, ranging from simple revenge to complicated blood feuds, can last for generations and lead to disaster. Nevertheless, as soon as one of the people involved consistently breaks the vicious circle that both sides have normally slipped into and chooses to take a leap of faith beyond their own shadow, they can rescue everyone concerned. In our example, Lisa may have to (let herself) eat humble pie for some time and be nice, friendly and obliging, even though at the beginning Franz will continue to revert to his program of being destructive time and time again. Here encouragement can be found in the general truth that it is often wiser to "give in" than to "give up".

The person who is wiser and more willing to get off their high horse, in this case Lisa, simply has to stay the course and stick to the program of "No matter what the other person does, I will simply give my best from now on" for long enough. This becomes easier if, for example, she thinks back to the early beginnings of the relationship, thereby reminiscing and connecting to their love in this early phase. While in a state of deep relaxation or trance, something like this is not difficult at all. In contrast, it is actually a very pleasant experience.[19] On top of this, it will help to clearly show once more just how pointless resistance actually is. Fighting against reality is as absurd as it is hopeless. There is only one thing that helps in such cases: accept what is, and ultimately even—as Byron Katie advises—love what is.

Lisa could recognize what a truly effective form of shadow therapy she has at her disposal if she chooses to take back her reproaches (b). In theory, she knows that the turnaround necessarily has to be true as well. "It's as easy as (a), (b), (c) (and (d)!) could become the decisive sentence for successful shadow hunters. As long as we still have feelings of resentment towards others: Let it all out (a)! But then take it all back (b) and use whatever the relevant topic is for your own growth! Anything that can help us to be daring enough to undertake this turnaround of responsibility and to manage to take the leap of faith beyond our own shadow is worth its weight in gold.

Following this, it will also do Lisa a lot of good to run through variant (c) and to thus indulge in another, usually very constructive form of therapy. This is because the realization: "I treat myself badly" (c) will soon lead her to notice this lack of self-respect and to put a stop to it. Instead, she will begin to get to know herself better and to treat herself honestly and decently.

---

19 The CD *Partner- und Beziehungsprobleme* (Partner and Relationship Problems*) is recommended for this.

In addition to the simple turnaround of guilt or responsibility (b), variant (c) also has the advantage of being within her own domain of influence. “Lisa treats Lisa badly”—That is something that Lisa can change.

In actual fact, when Lisa treats Franz badly, she also always treats herself badly at that same time. It is not at all possible to treat anyone else badly without doing something bad to yourself as well. We also find this very clearly formulated by Christ in the New Testament: “Truly I tell you, whatever you did not do for one of the least of these, you did not do for me. “. (Matthew 25:45)[20]

Consequently, Lisa could immediately take advantage of this great opportunity to do something good for herself by giving herself a gift, spoiling herself or giving herself her best—as she did for Franz as part of variant (b). Doing and giving our best represents a wonderful opportunity for ourselves. Those who give their best always give themselves a gift at the same time, no matter who they give their best to. It brings them joy as well as bringing joy to others in every moment and mobilizes amazing powers. While the turnaround of responsibility (b) seems to push us beyond our own powers, variant (c) can even serve as the start of a new era. Those who, in line with (c), have long since made peace with themselves can usually do so more easily with others.

At this point, there is still a final turnaround phase to be considered, namely: “Franz treats Franz badly” (d). This is, of course, also true and helps to make quite a number of things clear. Naturally, Franz treats himself badly if he treats his partner badly, since in doing so, he devalues his own integrity, thereby hurting his Self. His partner functions as a representative for his own female side. As a result, what he does to his partner is also always a blow to himself in the form of his anima, i.e. the feminine component of his soul (according to C. G. Jung), his princess (in line with the logic of fairy tales) or his better half (as

20 Holy Bible, New International Version®, NIV® Copyright ©1973, 1978, 1984, 2011 by Biblica, Inc.®

we say in everyday speech). Viewed the other way round, Lisa, with her reproaches against Franz (a), is naturally also delivering a blow to herself in the form of her male side, her animus and the masculine component of her soul, her inner hero, king's son or husband. In effect, she could give a lot to her inner better half by first giving it to Franz and could, in this way, carry out a considerable amount of psychotherapy on her own. This has the major advantage that it works while at the same time remaining entirely under her own control and costing nothing—except the overcoming of her initial resistance to making the effort. Over time, this simple form of therapy brings joyfulness and enthusiasm into the game of life. On top of this, the therapy is also contagious. Franz will quickly jump on board as well, and by giving to Lisa, will begin to enrich his better (female) half.

Even though these turnarounds can work miracles, there are, of course, limits to them. There are situations in which the shadow is acted out in physical abuse, such as beatings and rape, and is not limited to psychological abuse. In this case, what needs to be learned is resistance—both psychologically and physically. Sometimes the frog (from the fairy tale of *The Frog Prince*) needs to be flung against the wall instead of being kissed. The American expert when it comes to tracking down shadow, Byron Katie, also relies on this turnaround method. In addition to various questions that are used to invite people to engage in shadow work, Katie also employs this technique of converting reproaches into their opposites. In her books and workshops, Byron Katie illustrates her method with the help of many case studies that trace how the people involved manage to escape from the trap of projection into a life of taking responsibility for themselves. Such cases are a great opportunity that we cannot take advantage of often enough. The more such examples exist, the better. This is because the path of projection is wide and well-trodden, and in fact, should more accurately be described as an eight-lane superhighway. In contrast, the opposite pole, i.e. the taking back of responsibility for oneself can initially be likened to hacking one's way with a machete through an impenetrable mental jungle. Nevertheless, with every person who pushes their way through, and with every example that others experience, the path widens and becomes more accessible, and as such, is more clearly visible. To this end, here are also a few further examples:

The reproach made by a man towards his partner is: "She should stop continually blaming me for everything" (a) The turnaround is: "I should stop continually blaming her for everything" (b). This case also lends itself well to the pronoun game: "I should stop continually blaming myself" (c). And of course: "She should stop continually blaming herself" (d).

As always, (b) and (c) start off in the foreground, because (a) and (d) are not (yet) accessible to his influence. Nevertheless, the Law of Resonance ensures that these last two will also end up falling into place. With this first round of the game and the variants (b) and (c), the man experiences rapid success—something that he had failed to achieve during his many years of trying variant (a). For such a long time, he had complained to her directly and to all his friends about her. However, given that this is his reality, kicking up a storm against that same reality can achieve nothing. After he puts a stop to all of the reproaches towards his wife and instead sees through and minimizes his own constant complaints, his wife also begins to show more restraint in this respect. Their well-practised vicious circle becomes a spiral in the other direction. As success becomes more and more apparent, he eventually begins not only to refrain from reproaches, but even to pay her compliments, and in doing so, brings her former avalanche of reproaches to a complete standstill. Last but not least, he finally gets his long-awaited peace and quiet, and his partner also finds out how to take responsibility for her own life at his side. After he has removed the projection screen for her reproaches and accusations, she is forced to target her energy elsewhere and is able to direct it into more constructive activities. Her husband is proud of his success, but also of the fact that the therapy has managed to influence her so positively without her knowledge.

Another example: Mrs. M. accuses her husband P. of cheating on her with a younger woman, i.e. "He is cheating on me" as the variant (a). This accusation is a pretty standard one. Here the difficulty of the situation is heightened by the fact that Mr. P. is clearly younger than Mrs. M. and that she has therefore taken on a kind of mother role for him. She seeks help in counselling. She believes that he has been wanting to separate from her for a long time and that he is only staying with her out of gratitude, which he denies. The turnaround: "I'm cheating on him" (b) immediately brings her to tears, because it now dawns on her how she has been fooling herself and him for a long time. Of course, she has always been well aware of the large difference in age and the problems associated with it. In actual fact, she is not only his lover and mother, but also his therapist. Consequently, she is quite superior to him in many ways. Since she has always sensed the explosive potential of this for the relationship, she has always put on an act for him and has continually pretended to be less intelligent than she is—at least in his presence. By constantly selling herself short, she has been cheating on him and herself.

The variant (c): "I'm cheating on myself" raises even more issues, which she has long been aware of, but has consistently dodged facing. She has even started putting on an act for herself in order to save the relationship, in keeping with the motto: "Better the devil you know than the uncharted realm of freedom". Right from the very first consultation, she becomes far more self-aware and can therefore admit to being equally responsible. Consequently, it is easy for her to put an end to her accusations towards Mr P. once and for all. In addition, she abandons any further attempts to encourage him to engage in sexual activities and tries to be honest with herself and with him.

At the second consultation, Mr. P. turns up unannounced and is less understanding regarding her growing self-awareness than Mrs. M. was expecting. When all is said and done, he actually wants to keep her as a caregiver in the sense of being a mother figure as well as—admittedly not often, but every now and then—loving her as a sensual, erotic mother. At the same time, he wants to keep his younger and intellectually less- superior lover. Surprisingly, my client admits this very openly to him in the session, even though he would never have dared to formulate it this way explicitly himself. In fact, they live with this variant for some time until she falls in love with a partner who is "more equal" to her. Nevertheless, even at this point, she again falls into the "self-deception trap" and "cheats on" P. and herself by staying longer than she thinks she should, allegedly so as not to "hurt" him and leave him in a state of "defenceless vulnerability".

Mrs. M. again comes in for a consultation, and we repeat the game with the pronouns, with the result that she again decides to stop cheating on herself, and on her new and her old partner. In this way, the simple game with the pronouns, or in other words, with assigning responsibility, leads to a great step forward for her towards a new, more mature relationship. This also turns out to be the case even for P. Now that he is completely dependent on the relationship with the younger partner, this soon runs into problems that also lead to greater honesty.

Another example begins with Andrea's reproach towards Kurt: "You begrudge me everything, you are so stingy! (a). The turnaround: "I begrudge Kurt everything" (b) allows Andrea to recognize several painful truths, which cannot simply be rejected out of hand. The variant: "I begrudge myself everything" (c) shocks her at first, but evidence for this is soon found. That Kurt begrudges himself everything (d) has long been clear to her. Although this eases her suffering somewhat, it doesn't really improve either situation.

After playing the pronoun game, Andrea deliberately begins to pamper Kurt and to encourage him to treat himself more, while she takes more readily and also treats herself to much more. Tentatively, he learns to accept the former, and to her astonishment, has nothing against the latter. Over time, both find their way out of this stinginess trap. Andrea is amazed at just how happy she can be about her "therapy success", while Kurt starts to become more generous with himself every now and then. Those around them have been benefiting from both their growing tolerance and generosity for some time now. Andrea also discovers a further money problem of her own, which prevents her from enjoying common money unconditionally.

This small game with the pronouns can bring about great things and change a lot in a positive sense; its success stories could fill entire books on their own. Byron Katie's books do this and offer a wealth of (training) material and illustrative examples. Such games simply require a certain degree of courage and the willingness to be honest with oneself and to take responsibility for one's own life. In other words, they require the willingness to play with the pronouns in the reproachful sentences we direct at others and to shuffle these around. With this almost banal trick, we can get the lion's share of our shadow problems, namely our interpersonal problems, under control.

Practical Exercise

Take your time, and in your mind's eye, allow the people that you bear the most resentment towards in your life to appear. Take the person who first springs to mind—and have no fear, all of the others will get their turn.

Formulate your accusation against this person as variant (a). Play the turnaround game: first the reversal in variant (b), in which you take on the responsibility. Then variant (c) in which the issue stays with you, and finally, option (d) in which it shifts entirely to the other person. Perhaps you can later give the particular person tips, but only if the person involved invites you to do so. Repeat this highly important practical exercise with all those who you resent or reproach. And should a new case of resentment be added, simply play the pronoun game straightaway.

Examining blame-shifting with a magnifying glass

Whether you tend to blame yourself or others, it still remains projection. We can project our problems onto the outside world and create enemies. Alternatively, we can project them inwards onto our own organism and develop symptoms and disease patterns. We can shift the blame onto our own soul and sow feelings of guilt, which we then reap later in life. The assigning of blame in whatever form is a crucial shadow topic.

In confronting the shadow, the whole point is to bring problems particularly close to oneself instead of pushing them as far away from oneself as possible. It is important to realize that, , as with all meaningful shadow work, both the turnaround process and the alternation game with the pronouns serve to bring responsibility (back) to ourselves. Ultimately, it is necessary to make a conscious shift from being the poor victim to acting as a self-responsible perpetrator. In this context, the very concept of a “perpetrator” loses its negative connotation. This proactive complicity allows us to develop into dynamic and decisive people who take responsibility for our own lives, and as such, we then become co-creators, in a positive sense, of our own path in life. If we understand blame as a debt we owe to wholeness, it becomes even easier.

The complaint: “I hate being constantly given the blame for everything,” should be familiar to many of us. Of course, accepting outstanding dues, as far as blame is concerned, which some people tend to take upon themselves, is practical for the people around them, because then the guilt is taken care of. This corresponds to the old scapegoat policy that was followed by early tribal societies and which we can read about in the Bible: the people chose a ram or goat, thrust all blame upon it, then chased it away into the desert, thus freeing themselves of all guilt. And of course, this is correct: As soon as someone takes all of the blame upon him- or herself or even actively draws it towards him- or herself, the rest of us are relieved of the burden. Nevertheless, at the same time, this hinders the development of such groups and communities. In this respect, the ritual of choosing a symbolic scapegoat instead, which has been handed down to us by history, seems to be the much better way.

Although blame and guilt have their place in social life, in our modern society we do not value such scapegoat rituals highly enough. As a result, blame ends up being scattered all over the place instead, and little distinction is made between responsibility and blame. Everyone needs to be constantly on their guard to avoid being unfairly lumped with blame. On the whole, this makes the general mood in modern society anxious and tense. Many of its members live in constant fear of the blame/responsibility complex and are always on the run from it.

Since the game with the pronouns is so comprehensive and can be applied to practically all aspects of modern society, we can save ourselves the effort of unravelling all of the complex psychological interconnections each time. It is enough to simply play the game of working through the three other variants (b, c, d) with the pronouns right from the very first reproach (a). This playful method for taking back the projections will soon change your life in a noticeable, and in fact, drastic way. There is no need to worry, however, that life will get boring when there is no-one else to blame. On the contrary, you will gain considerably more responsibility, which makes life more exciting. The ancient philosopher Epictetus says in effect the following: uneducated people who are having a rough time seek the blame for it in their environment; philosophical beginners who are having a rough time seek the blame for it in themselves. In such situations, however, truly educated people do not seek guilt either from outside or from within.

If you stop putting the blame on yourself and others and instead take responsibility for yourself, you will experience a kind of miracle. This is because, in accordance with the Law of Resonance, those around you must also eventually stop putting the blame on you. In this way, you will continue to develop towards a life that is free of blame and guilt and that feels incomparably pleasant. Looking back, the former familiar process of pushing sin back and forth will seem downright ridiculous.

Often, the original reproach in variant (a) is not actually even really true at all. This stems from the tendency of the intellectual left hemisphere of our brain to overgeneralize, exaggerate, blur, and rationalize certain positions and spin these together so that the ego's point of view, which is so narrow because it is so limited, becomes more bearable.

Practical Exercise

Examine some of your favourite reproaches from the past with the same magnifying glass that you have used to badger yourself and those around you. Find out whether variant (a) even corresponded to reality at all. If you happen to discover that that was not actually the case, you can always resort to a direct apology after the fact. Relieving yourself of your "burden of guilt" will release tension more quickly and be the wind beneath your wings that will uplift you.

Record your impressions in your shadow diary—and apply this practical exercise in general at all times.

In the Stoa, the doctrine of wisdom that was just quoted, Epictetus advocates not seeking guilt anywhere. In contrast, according to the Catholic biblical doctrine, we all share in the hereditary guilt or Original Sin that arose through eating from the Tree of Knowledge of Good and Evil. Consequently, in entering this world of opposites, a debt in the form of guilt entered the (Christian) world at the same time. The advantage of this perspective can lie in admitting to ourselves that we all have our *failings*.

With every decision we make, we *fail* to choose something else that would be needed for wholeness. Realizing this could make genuinely begging the pardon of others much easier.

To truly beg the pardon of others, we would have to take a leap of faith beyond our own shadow in the truest sense of the word, which in our context is a very healing exercise. A deeply felt "I beg your pardon" is often successful and actually leads to forgiveness. This relieves the soul in a decisive way and heals it in the sense of becoming more whole.

In addition, fundamental feelings of guilt, such as those derived from the Original Sin, could remind us of what we still "owe" to wholeness or to life or our life task. "Sins", or in other words "debts", can therefore only be settled by a conscious return to wholeness itself, which in accordance with Christian theology, was already lost in paradise. In keeping with this, it is our task in this world of contrasts to overcome this loss and to reverse the separation. But this is only possible through developing ourselves further. Only when we unite our Ego with our shadow in the sense of self-realization does this original guilt end and we then return to innocence.

Shadow diary

How easy do I find it to forgive? What role has blame played in how I was raised? in my life? Am I able to praise well and easily? How willing am I to be grateful?

Please record your answers in your shadow diary.

The world as our mirror

Are circumstances to blame?

The simple method for dealing with shadow in interpersonal conflicts that was already described above, namely the game with the pronouns, may seem somewhat astonishing. However, as soon as two people have an issue with each other, this will swing back and forth between them. It is only various firmly-entrenched and highly-habitualised power-play structures that allow us to overlook this. No-one can ever be jealous or hurtful by themselves. Nevertheless, when the issues at hand are not simply interpersonal issues, but instead involve objects and circumstances or whole societies that are totally "overshadowed" by reproaches, more knowledge is necessary to see through it all. Those who blame the economic system, the government, taxes, the health system, the media or the weather for their lack of success are stuck in a more difficult trap. A few examples may illustrate this: "I grew up in an area far from the sea and without any lakes and ponds, and no-one travelled much back then," says an elderly patient. "That's why I never learned to swim and was terribly ashamed of it later. As time went by, things got worse and worse, because swimming pools sprang up everywhere. But now it was already too late for me. Then they even started installing those terrible swimming pools in all of the hotels, and from then on, there was practically nowhere I could go without embarrassing myself. That's why all of my relationships eventually failed or actually didn't really get going in the first place."

A young man reports: "When I was fourteen, I knocked out my front teeth in an accident and then had to wear false teeth like an old man. I was so embarrassed that I didn't dare kiss a girl, let alone share a bedroom or a bathroom with a woman. As a result, I could never have a longer relationship and never be happy. This of course had an effect on my job and on everything in general."

A further example displaying an amazing chain of projections: "Because I didn't have a high school diploma, I couldn't study, and that's why I didn't get the job of my choice. As a result, I was never able to find the right partner, and so I have never known true love. I also never earned enough money to be able to afford what I wanted. That's why I can't help but consider my life a failure and yet I can't help it at all."

If, as a therapist, you trace back these kinds of projection chains, the guilt is usually always shifted back further and further. In the last case ("Because I didn't have a high school diploma ..."), the patient added that there was no hope of her passing the final examination because a teacher let her fail "out of sheer meanness". In the first of the above cases, the initiative and courage to face the challenge of swimming are in the shadow—and thus an aggression issue is at stake. This is remarkably often the case at the beginning of such chains, since the energy underlying the principle of aggression is also the same "kickoff energy" needed for every beginning. In the consciousness of the patient, however, it is the (lack of) access to water that is to blame. Fittingly, water corresponds to the soul. Anyone who has never had access to the soul element will build up psychological shadow, especially if, as in this case, that person takes the inability to swim as a reason for the failure of her relationships and ultimately of her own life.

In the second case, the issue of aggression is also addressed, this time in a concrete form with respect to the teeth. No longer having real weapons in your mouth as a young man certainly puts you at a disadvantage. Nevertheless, the issues of self-assertion, courage and energy could be worked on and learned about in other forms in order to still be able to stand up for oneself, instead of simply pushing this aspect deep into the shadow domain. In the case given here, it serves as a smokescreen for letting the whole topic of relationships fail. Where aggression, energy and strength are not brought into the game of life, of course, not much gets going.

In the third case story, the mention of "school", "teacher" and "examination" at first points towards the principle of communication and mediation, which obviously came up too short. In this case as well, however, initiative and self-assertion have also slipped into the domain of shadow. The simple turnaround strategy from the pronoun game can be applied very well here: "The teacher did not like me", is the original accusation (a). The equally certain turnaround is: "I did not like the teacher" (b). This is, at the very least, just as probable, and in any case, far more productive, because she could have changed something about that, which was not the case for the initial situation.

If she had worked on her aversion to the teacher, he might—through the process of resonance—have gradually taken on a more positive attitude towards her over time. It is possible that even just polite friendliness would have been enough.

At the same time, the other two variants would also have been helpful. "I didn't like myself" (c)—the fact that she didn't try to repeat her final year of high school speaks for this variant. And also the variant (d) is probable: "The teacher didn't like himself".

Maybe that's why he was a bad teacher and felt dissatisfied and why he was so tough on a girl who didn't like herself either. And even if the main reason had been the initially unjust teacher, her only chance would have been to start with the two variants that she could actually influence: namely, her aversion towards the teacher (b) and towards herself (c). Ultimately, it all comes down to being willing to accept the very simple challenge of pointing the finger at oneself. This offers by far the best and overall the most excellent opportunities.

When it comes to projecting onto circumstances and things, it is very helpful to grasp what the underlying theme is in order to see who or what is being declared guilty on a deeper level of reality. If the non-swimmer had recognized the spiritual aspect associated with the element of water and cared more about her soul and everything spiritual in life, a better way (out) would certainly have been revealed to her. If the toothless young man had recognized the principle of aggression underlying his issues and worked on that on all possible other levels, his problem would also have been solvable. If he had thrown commitment and fighting spirit, decisiveness and courage and the fire of his young enthusiasm into the mix to tip the scales in his favour, he would certainly have been successful on the sports field; his strong body seemed to indicate this. Then he would certainly also have received offers of interest for relationships. In addition, time—to the same extent that it worked against the non-swimmer—would have worked in his favour with the development and provision of continually improved dental prostheses all the way up to implants. The decisive factor would have been finding access to his problem, toothlessness on many different levels.

Meditation

Read Meditations 1 & 6 aloud to yourself.

Afterwards, allow yourself sufficient time to let the meditation come to a harmonious close. Then return to the here and now by taking a deep breath that connects you again with polarity in our world of opposites. Re-orient yourself consciously in space by stretching and moving your body, and in time, by taking a look at your watch.

Repeat the exercise as often as you wish with different projections onto other situations, circumstances and things, and entrust your initial results to your shadow diary.

Complaining achieves nothing

While on a cruise, one of the guests explained to me how he was attempting to cash in on the trip with the aid of blame projection. At first, I had thought he was an artist because he was photographing the strangest of minor details. On the other hand, he seemed extremely stuffy and conservative, and he was taking the pictures with a cheap camera. He willingly let me in on his secret: he was a specialist in the lodging of complaints and right from the very first day of travel, he began to register everything that he could use as the basis for compensation claims. He proudly reported that he was almost always reimbursed at least a quarter and sometimes even half of the price of the trip as a gesture of goodwill. He was completely perplexed when I explained that this was in effect actually a bad deal: while he ruined the trip for himself one hundred percent every time, at best he only got fifty percent of the money back.

Those who spend their whole lives banking on blame projections seem to me to be acting in a similar way. Although they can be 100 percent certain about ending up in a state of depressing frustration, shifting the blame does not help to reduce the burden of their existence to any significant degree. No matter how you choose to look at it, this is an extremely poor deal and a miserable outlook on life. The following example of a shadow analysis may further illustrate the hopelessness of such lines of complaint: "My wife has found someone else. She is being unfaithful and inconsiderate; her behaviour is unchristian and embarrassing for me. She should not be doing that." This situation would bring the vast majority of husbands into resistance with reality and, vice versa, most wives. Nevertheless, many couples live in precisely this situation for a long time and poison each other's lives without drawing the obvious consequences. Even if they do eventually draw these and separate, their reproaches often persist and poison life beyond the divorce. In the worst-case scenario, the reproaches are then carried into the lives of their shared children and so end up burdening the next generation as well.

Struggling against the reality of a relationship, no matter how depressing that reality may be, in the form of reproaches or demands therefore offers less-than-promising prospects. In contrast, recognizing reality is very easy, because obviously, in fact even by her own admission, she, the wife, has another found someone else. It is important to acknowledge this. It is a fact and storming against it will do nothing to change it. Most probably the other relationship is offering her something that is important to her and that she, seemingly, is not getting anywhere else, and in any case, certainly not from her husband. The consultation enabled him to realize that, firstly, insisting on his position would, in all likelihood, not bring her back, and secondly, he would also deprive himself of all the opportunities he still had available to him in his own life. For months he had clung tightly to his reproachful demands, but this had shown no effect. His wife felt unable to come back to him (on an erotic level) and this was causing dramatic suffering in his life as a result.

Let's deal with the original complaint in more detail: "My wife has found someone else. She should not be doing that. She is being unfaithful and inconsiderate. It is unchristian and humiliating for me ... She must stop it immediately and apologize to me" (a). When I asked him to undertake the turnaround of responsibility with regard to these statements, a lot of interesting things came out that shed considerable light on the whole affair. Playing the game with the pronouns was again the key to initiating a turnaround in both his actions and his thinking: "I have found someone else; I should not be doing that" (b). In actual fact, he had had an affair twice before and still keenly felt a strong sense of injustice, as well as having a very bad conscience. Even though he had never freely admitted to his indiscretion, she knew about it. In retrospect, he still felt himself to have been unfaithful and inconsiderate, for he had even become angry and lashed out at her when she had confronted him with her suspicions. Unlike his wife, he found the whole thing to be very unchristian and immoral himself, because he was a devout Catholic. As such, it was quite obviously actually his own problem that he was accusing her of. He freely admitted to the sense of humiliation being totally his own issue. Back then, his wife had been angry and upset and had asked him to end the affair. He had done so—the first time at least—extremely reluctantly, bowing to her pressure and that of his religious beliefs. He had never apologized and asked for forgiveness, although he had had the strong feeling that he should have done so. Nevertheless, since he hadn't admitted to anything, it had, of course, been impossible to do so. As a result, he`d wound up well and truly stuck with a huge pile of guilt. By denying the truth, he had blocked off the path to an apology by himself. In contrast, his wife had already apologized at the very first confrontation, but did not really end the other relationship. She did, at least, however, admit to continuing to see the other man.

His belief that she had to stop the relationship immediately was obviously naive and definitely not true at all. For she didn't stop, and it was this reality that was tormenting him. He continued to stick resolutely to his demands, but had no power whatsoever to enforce them. In contrast, his now hopeless insistence on an idealized state that had long since ceased to be true only made him even more aware of his own unhappiness. There was no way for him to force her to end the relationship with the other guy. His only available option was for them to separate, which he definitely did not want to do.

The fact that he was getting the problems of his own psyche reflected in his wife and her situation and was thus experiencing his own shadow became clear to him in the course of the conversation. He also finally understood that it was actually ridiculous to insist on something that simply wasn't true. His wife didn't have to return to him at all. Little by little, he began to understand that he was only harming himself and their relationship even further. Even more important, however, was working out how his second affair had come about. The reason was to be found in the other woman, who had fascinated him more, or at least, had fascinated him in a new way. Everything was more exciting with her instead of things being taken for granted and taking place within a well-worn rut. He had felt young and full of energy again. He had then noticed exactly the same thing about his wife, and this had aroused his suspicion. In contrast to him, however, she had admitted to everything immediately.

In our conversation, it now became apparent how he had also admitted to his affair, even if only indirectly. It had been small slipups that had aroused her attention. In this way, he had let her in on his secret by betraying himself—unconsciously. The covert reason for this was that he wanted to get rid of the extramarital affair because he could not accept it internally.

To the extent that he recognized himself and his own shadow in his wife and what she was experiencing and then faced up to this reality, his condemnation of her became noticeably milder. He could now put himself in her shoes and thus developed something akin to compassion. When, soon after, he confessed his own two relationships to her retrospectively and apologized to her, this act of honesty helped to win her back a little. When, on the basis of the psychotherapy sessions that he had begun, he also began to consciously integrate everything that had fascinated him about his love affairs and put them into action in his home life, he gradually won her back more and more.

His realization that he had simply been accusing her of what he been rejecting in himself and thus actually accusing himself of, gave him strength and courage once again and endowed their relationship with new energy and hope. Both experienced their marriage afterwards as better and more fulfilling. The reason for this is that honesty always acts as a turn-on and shedding light on the shadow even more so. Through the integration of this experience, and above all, the integration of other new aspects into their relationship life, they had both grown; their respective affairs alone had by no means brought this about. He had shed light on a large chunk of his shadow and had learned to be more honest with himself and with her, as well as becoming more broadminded and open, which she found very attractive.

As I almost always do after such experiences, in which people have made the leap of faith beyond their own shadow, I try to seize the golden opportunity to encourage the people concerned not to be content with just this one example, but to extend this successful concept to the rest of their life. In this case, the client immediately came up with this same idea by himself and asked if I could perhaps help him in a similar way with his main rival in the company. Naturally, he managed to achieve this himself by using the same mechanism of doing shadow analysis. He now knew that whatever accusations he had towards his work colleague (a) also applied in this case to himself (b).

Talking about others behind their backs was equally a habit of his, especially as far as this "guy" was concerned, but supposedly only as a form of self-defense. Just like my client, this guy was continually doing his best to not only make a good impression on their mutual boss, but to actually outdo his rival as often as possible. When it came to his colleague, he naturally had no problem recognizing this as opportunism and sucking up to his superiors. After my client finally saw through all of this and stopped acting this way of his own free will, the relationship improved "all by itself". From this point on, the two of them even managed to have more relaxed conversations with one another, and the patient experienced the magic of the Law of Resonance. Now, many years later, he and his wife can look back on a life lived in a far more conscious way in the light of *the Laws of Fate*, including the concepts of Polarity and Shadow. His wife even imparts this knowledge, which liberated them both, to others in the sense of a resonance field of "contagious good health".

Even back then, the patient had already asked me to write a little book about these simple tricks that had helped him so much. At the time, this seemed to me to be too simplistic and too lacking in originality. Could two such simple statements like "Face the truth and you'll be free" and "Take back your projections" possibly be enough to fill a whole book? Both reminders seemed almost too banal to me. Not only were they lacking in originality, they had not even originated from me. In the second reminder, the Christian commandment to "love your enemies" shines through all too clearly. In actual fact, our symptoms are our enemies. These can appear internally in the form of illness symptoms and externally in the form of opponents, different types of resistance and whatever makes us uncomfortable. We also find them in our complaints, wish lists and suggestions for improvement. All of these lead us to greater freedom, and this book is aims to help with this process.

Shadow diary

How can I extend the knowledge I have gained so far on dealing with shadow to other domains and issues?

Record your thoughts and answers in writing

Bullying as an example

If you end up being a victim of bullying, the most effective and simplest anti-bullying therapy is to stop talking badly about others. According to the Law of Resonance, the other side will then also stop talking badly about you. Of course, this approach does not prevent the victim from actively defending him- or herself in line with the Law of Polarity. The basic reproach is: "They are talking badly about me" (a). The turnaround already tells us a lot: "I am talking badly about them" (b). But also: "I talk or think badly about myself" (c), and: "They think badly about themselves" (d).

To date, every victim of bullying or slander that I have known—including myself—also talked badly about others themselves or at the very least had bad thoughts about them. In my own case, of course, I could immediately find the connection between the slander directed at me and my often harsh criticisms directed against orthodox medicine and its followers. I had always thought it didn't count in the same way if I did so without mentioning specific names, but it does.

When we actively seek to confront our own shadow rather than trying to fight against the outside world, it is easy to be successful using what we have worked out so far as a basis. The first step is to give up our resistance to reality. No matter how that reality appears to us, we must learn to accept it exactly as it is as the prerequisite for any further development. Reality keeps on working, whether we accept it or not, and it has brought us to precisely this point in our development. This is the only truth that we can build upon. Regardless of what we have pieced together in terms of our own assumed truths, we must measure our own mosaic of truths against this reality and, if necessary, bid farewell to our preferred truths in favour of the truth of what is.

The second step is to recognize our projections for what they really are. This step already overlaps to some extent with the first step, because our projections include the "yarns" that we have spun together to help us to see the world as it suits the ego. They allow us to remain in the role of the "poor victim" without taking on any responsibility for ourselves. The world is then to blame for everything, and we can feel miserable and totally in the right about it at the same time.

The withdrawal of such projections, in contrast, involves assuming responsibility for what is. No-one else matters at this point. We may no longer be in the right, but at any rate, we are now responsible, and we may still feel bad, perhaps even worse in the beginning. However, there is hope for us once again if we face up to this responsibility for ourselves.

In the process of doing this, finding the right level of existence for taking on responsibility may become a problem. Fate is usually more than willing to show us the problem and the underlying principle that it belongs to. At the same time, however, it typically presents us with the more considerable challenge of finding the respective level of existence that corresponds to us personally. When I experience malicious gossip, it means that I talk or at least think badly about others as well. Which domain this applies to, however, is something that I have to find out on my own by being extremely open and honest with myself and sometimes even by enlisting outside help? Often it may be the case that I do not think badly about the same person who is talking badly about me. In addition, with the passing of time and our increasing awareness of life, minor transgressions will be brought to our attention by means of more formidable external events. What else can Fate to do when our own projections become more and more sophisticated and more cleverly concealed? It has to bring out the heavier artillery, and we then have the ever more challenging task of successfully working out the various translation steps to find the appropriate level that applies to us.

Of course, we can choose to feel unjustly treated again, and to judge the reaction of Fate as disproportionate. Nevertheless, this would again simply be a complaint to the Universe or a projection. Alternatively, we could instead choose to feel honored that Fate has chosen to put so much effort into giving us a helpful shove in the right direction towards making the all-important leap of faith beyond our own shadow.

Bullying is a particularly good example for understanding the nature of shadow analysis and projection. People suffering from bullying come to others seeking help and simply want the bullying to stop in the external world. In this phase, they would prefer to have the aid of the police to restore order and would like to see those who are talking badly about them severely punished. As soon as it becomes clear to them how much the problem lies within them, they typically react reluctantly all the way to total disbelief and counter this with "Yes, but ..." rationalizations. They believe that they have many good reasons and even real proof that the problem lies with other people and in the external world.

Nevertheless, this is the secret behind every projection: it seems true and genuine without actually being so. Without a doubt, projection is by far the most widespread delusion. Those affected become totally entangled in their own homespun fabrication of reality. They seem totally wrapped up in a cocoon of rationalizations and pseudo-justifications. Any other delusion will also seem true and genuine to someone who is delusional. In extreme cases, it can take a long time until the delusion is really seen through.

In the wonderful film *A Beautiful Mind*, Russell Crowe, in the role of Nobel Prize winner John Forbes Nash, fights a heroic battle against characters from his own delusional imagination. Fortunately, the delusion of projection is not nearly as deep-rooted and tough to get rid of as psychotic delusions are. However, under special circumstances, such projections can also take on a similar delusional character in a psychiatric sense. In the everyday sense of the word, these projections are already "delusional", because they are both unrealistic and unreal with respect to reality, although they seem so extremely real to those affected by them.

The task in terms of therapy is not to convince the person concerned of the opposite. That is difficult, if not impossible. Instead, it is enough to win them over for the pursuit of their own self-development. Since there is usually no possibility to change the situation in the external world, such "victims" can occasionally be motivated to give this a try. In some cases, the "victims" can also be convinced of how unrealistic their attitude is. "That (simply) cannot be (true); the situation must stop immediately", are typical sentiments that are expressed. And yet, it is true and it does not stop. In most cases, it has actually been going on for quite a while. And since that is exactly what those affected have experienced, it is easy to convince them of the essential truth of this.

We can feel sorry for ourselves and complain about something, but we usually cannot change it in the external world. On the other hand, we can always change ourselves and our attitude. Since it is usually the only thing at all that we can do immediately, this carries a lot of persuasive power and has the best chances of success. Even in those instances—rare enough as they are—in which we can change something in the external world, the results are often not particularly good, and by no means comparable, with the results of inner shadow work. If the patient whose wife was cheating on him had managed to compel or even coerce her into giving up the relationship using pressure, threats, blackmail, or even just by giving her a bad conscience, they would never have experienced the same sense of relief and feelings of joy after getting back together afterwards. If the same patient had had the power to dismiss his rival at his workplace, "the problem" would have been solved initially. However, his own inner problem would certainly have then moved onto someone else; it would have simply been a question of time. As soon as one problematic case has been driven away, a new one arrives—this phenomenon is experienced in groups, departments and entire companies time and time again. Alternatively, the potential energy of the problem ends up spread over several people who had previously been spared. Attempts to solve the problem in the external world merely shift this potential energy elsewhere, internal solutions resolve it.

Basically, shadow analysis entails the unravelling of such attempts to shift responsibility, or more precisely, the disentanglement of the tangled web of confusion that has arisen as a result. The courageous game with the pronouns is the greatest help in dealing with interpersonal issues. It is easy to try out each new variation and to examine deep within our soul whether this statement is perhaps truer and more helpful than our original reproach or complaint. In addition, it is enormously supportive to direct the appropriate questions to one's own soul while in a state of deep relaxation, and preferably in trance.

Film Meditation

Watch the film *A Beautiful Mind* with an attitude of meditative relaxation. As you do so, consider any delusional ideas of your own that you simply haven't got as worked up about in such a strong way. Are you aware of how persistent shadow is—especially your own—and how long and complex the process of confronting it is, but also how worthwhile and rewarding? Once again, use the end of the film as the starting point for your own follow-up review in the image world of your own soul.

Inner Images—Allowing the soul to speak

Recognizing our inner reality

The language of the soul is one of images. It is through the use of this language that we can expect to find the best solutions when it comes to shadow work. At the same time, this language uncovers the simplest access point to the treasures of the shadow realm. As such, it grants us entry to the unbounded riches of our inner world, including those of the unconscious, which of course, can also only be experienced through images.

Spiritual energy, which in all cultures is connected with the element of water, flows in a perpetual stream, just like the creeks, rivers and currents of nature, infusing our entire being in the same way that water does in nature. Just as life cannot exist without water; without images, there can be no understanding of the soul. The fertility and creative power of the soul are as boundless as these same forces in nature. In an incessant flow, the soul creates and processes inner images on every level of our existence.

The world of the soul is connected with the feminine at the deepest level. In this sense, the image-based language of the soul is actually our original "mother" tongue and should be seen as preceding the language of the intellect. It is high time we learned to speak and understand it once again. Obviously, those who truly want to comprehend the way of life in another country, in another culture need to immerse themselves in its unique linguistic imagery and to make use of the language it entails. In exactly the same way, those who really want to get to know their soul need to delve into the image worlds of the soul.

This special system of image production is like the digestive system of the soul. In a constant stream, we absorb external images via our senses, both beautiful images and terrifying ones. With these, we nourish the realm of our soul. Just like water, the soul in its archetypically-feminine nature unwaveringly absorbs everything. In this way, it (or perhaps better "she") becomes the catchment basin for our collective experiences—not just for our individual experiences, but also for our collective experiences and even for the experiences of human evolution in general. Ceaselessly, the soul absorbs, digests and reconstitutes, structures, transforms and sets impressions, memories, conscious and unconscious perceptions and realizations in motion.

Even those who have not yet had any experience with image therapy still come into daily contact—or perhaps we should more accurately say, nightly contact—with the ocean of images of their soul. Every night, the soul reminds us in our dreams of her existence—a phenomenon which we modern humans find so difficult to grasp. It is here that she shows us how powerful she is in comparison with the minuteness of our daily consciousness. Nevertheless, we much prefer to identify ourselves with the latter, because this creates the illusion of having control over our lives, and even over our fate. In dreams, however, we can no longer rely on the coordinates of this earthly, material existence, which supposedly offers us a sense of security. Space and time are barrier gates that the realm of the soul knows nothing about. With natural abandon, she oversteps boundaries, breaks through them or simply dissolves them into thin air. In this way, a space of freedom is created that is as limitless as the universe. Everything is possible; security and certainty become lost in the ocean of boundless opportunities. The Persian poet and sufi Saadi of Shiraz put it into the following way: "Deep in the sea, there are countless treasures, but if you seek safety, it is on the shore."

Every dream represents our inner truth, and our reality as it is, and not as we would like it to be. Every dream can therefore be taken as a message from the soul, designed to offer us other meaningful viewpoints and insights. In this respect, dreams and their content are for the most part free of value judgements. Dreams merely show; they do not say what the dreamer must do. Above all, they show what actually *is* in the current existential situation of the dreamer. At the same time, they remain incorruptibly bound by the inner truth of the dreamer. They reveal what is—without evaluation, judgement or criticism. In this sense, they were seen as important by practically all archaic cultures. The "Dreamtime" of the Aborigines—the original inhabitants of Australia—is merely the example that is most well known to us.

It could be said that dreams and inner images show a pure form of reality. Here there are no conditions imposed, no consequences demanded. That role is left to our day-to-day consciousness. Since language is a servant of the intellect, dreams and inner images cannot be translated one-to-one into words. The language of dreams is one of symbols—and, as such, does not involve one-to-one unambiguous interpretations, but instead many-to-one ambiguities, since each symbol carries a great number of different levels of meaning in itself. What happens on the level of inner images in dreams, therapy or active imagination is far more analogical than logical. Even one and the same image has a slightly different correspondence and analogy for each person. For example, the symbol of the heart might represent the feeling of love and openness for one person, but fear and pain for another, depending on which feelings have become coupled to that symbol.

Symbols, images, and especially inner images have their own powerful effect. When it comes to great visions, we sense this force very clearly, but this is also true for shadow-related dreams, for example, when a nightmare leaves us feeling emotionally off- balance long after awakening.

Just how powerful the effect of inner images can be is evident in the original meaning of the word "imagination". Originally, it referred to the formation of an image, both in the sense of an illusion or delusion, as well as in the sense of something being pictured (internally) or in effect "conjured up". In this respect, it is no coincidence that, in the word "imagination", we find the word "magi(c)". The term is derived from Old Persian and designated the task that members of the priest caste fulfilled in acting as spiritual guides for the soul. These "magicians" had to interpret dreams, banish evil (inner) spirits, call upon good and healing powers; in short, they accompanied human souls on their dangerous life and developmental path between heaven and earth. In doing so, they were fully aware of the power and force of our inner reality and were masters of symbols and imagery.

The western world has disregarded this part of reality for a long time now. In line with logic, analysis, and left-hemisphere perceptions of reality, the "magical" worldview of the soul is viewed with derision. It is only small children who have been allowed to entertain this kind of perception for a brief period of time when, in play, they step into their fantasy world and experience it as real. Nevertheless, such a powerful component of reality cannot simply be pushed aside. What has been repressed is starting to become pressing. The long-disregarded realm of the soul is once again making its presence known in the form of rampant psychological problems that are now of considerable relevance for society. This has led to a certain extent to the resurrection of the old Persian priest caste in the form of modern psychotherapists. At the same time, it has become more and more apparent just how little the dimension of the soul can be addressed using analysis and left-hemispheric technology.

Guided meditations, dream interpretations, and the process of conscious imagining are now once again opening up more and more new territory for the soul. In a world and era, in which creativity as a source of innovation is in high demand, we are now turning our thoughts back to the roots of creative power. Imagination, our inner ability to visualize, is the cradle for the creative energy within us, and can be recognized particularly clearly in all forms of the visual arts, poetry, literature and music. In addition, when it comes to almost all ground-breaking scientific discoveries, imagination has also played a part. Bold scientific minds like Albert Einstein have always freely admitted this. The unlimited space generated by the freedom of the soul contains reality in its entirety—in its luminary, creative aspects, but also in its dark, fear-inducing dimensions. »*Per aspera ad astra*« (through the darkness to the light)—this requirement shows the underlying pattern of the path of spiritual development towards the source of creativity, towards the treasure chamber of inner riches. In Greek mythology, there is an archetypal figure, a god, which in western thinking, essentially represents the embodiment of a primordial pattern or archetype. The myth genre is, in actual fact, nothing more than the original alphabet of the image and symbol-based language of the soul, joined together in words and stories.

Myths are the inner expression and representation of primordial patterns or archetypes. In Greek mythology, which is of special importance for our "western" soul, the god Hades-Pluto rules over the dead or the shadow kingdom of the same name. He therefore is synonymous with the shadow kingdom of our soul, and for everything that we are not aware of, for what is in the dark, for what we've repressed, including possible "skeletons in the closet". In mythology, it is the heroes who are the only ones to enter Hades while still alive and to leave it again with rich rewards. They stand for those people who have set out to resolutely follow the path of development. Their hero's journey corresponds to the psychological individuation process, the path to oneself, and ultimately to unity, to God or whatever the final destination is named.

We ordinary heroes and heroines also follow this same path in our own way and at our own pace. We can choose to explore our own realm of shadows, or in other words, our personal Hades, consciously and of our own free will, for example, in the form of psychotherapy. However, we are often dragged there instead against our will by crises, illnesses and blows of Fate. In any case, our task, as soon as we find ourselves there, whether of our own volition or not, is to allow light into the darkness. It is necessary to have the courage to look into the darkness of our soul, in a way that is free of judgement, much like a mentally-sound child listens to a fairy tale. Here the wicked witch also has an undisputed place and is a central part of the fateful events that take place and the overall path of development.

It is in the darkest depths of the Earth that the most precious jewels lie, guarded by Hades Pluto, who was also revered as the god of (inner) riches, the source of all creative power. As already mentioned, our greatest inner treasures and talents are hidden in the shadow realm of our soul. They are waiting there patiently, ready to be unearthed. The easiest and most effective way to enter the picture realm of the soul is to use the technique of conscious imagination. This requires a phase of relaxation, which leads to a sense of calmness and *release*, because the archetypally-feminine soul requires serenity in order to allow her essence to unfold. She will elude any form of active *doing* or *making* in the sense of wanting to achieve something. Once this state of passive allowance has arisen, the therapist can, through the use of a symbolic image, then offer the patient the entrance gate into the realm of the soul. In this realm of unlimited possibilities, we can be sure that a *wonder*ful journey will begin that will allow the patient not only to recognize, but also to strongly feel and experience his or her inner riches at a deeper level. With each new entry, gaining access becomes easier, and our ability to creatively handle the problems we have brought with us gets better and better. It is in this environment that real solutions are born, especially to the extent that the person seeking them succeeds in taking note of and considering noteworthy whatever thought first arises. There is a special magic and charm associated with the first moment and thought that cannot be treasured highly enough. In this respect, the first thought that arises during our excursions while using the meditations should be assigned decisive significance.

Experience with this method in therapy settings has shown on numerous occasions just how clear and simple real solutions are. However, our complicated intellectual need to take action and an oversupply of arguments and rationalizations often blocks us from seeing those solutions. Time and time again, it is exhilarating and awe-inspiring to experience how the immeasurable wonders of the soul are revealed in these images. No two journeys of adventure into the soul will ever be exactly alike. The world of images is limitless, and everything is an image. Every life is a giant painting, a jigsaw puzzle, whose individual pieces are longing to be assembled to form a grand picture of each individual life. This is our mission in life. In this respect, almost all of the practical exercises in this book can be used to find individual pieces that are missing in your own life puzzle. Whether in the process of doing this, it is always clear to you on the intellectual level what this actually means in each case is at first secondary. The images are effective in and of themselves. The magic of transformation is contained within them.[21] It is in this sense that the meditation *Shadow work**, which devotes itself to the topic of this book within the world of inner imagery of the soul, can be understood.

---

21 For many topics, CDs with relevant guided meditations are available, in particular, also the CD *Shadow work**. Please refer to the list of references.

Dealing with our own shadow

The more often you find yourself in the situation of being perceived differently than how you see yourself and want to be seen, the less you truly know yourself and the more important a confrontation with your own shadow becomes. Friends and impartial observers are important in the showdown with our own shadow, since the ego is an unbelievably ingenious saboteur. While the ego—just as it doing right now—may pretend to be following along with great interest, it is actually secretly carrying clever rationalisations and excuses in its arsenal. For that reason, you shouldn't hesitate to ask for a second and third opinion, just as we are gradually learning to do in medicine in relation to all central questions of physical health. In this case, we are dealing with our mental and spiritual health, and for those aspects, further opinions are just as important. The Bible tells us that we can see the shadow of others far better than our own, because we recognize the "splinter" in the eye of another, but fail to recognize the entire "log" in our own. For this reason, when doing shadow work, we need to obtain the support of others.

What is decisive for the success of shadow integration is whether you succeed in preventing your ego from sabotaging the entire enterprise, for example, by constantly justifying your own behaviour and by nipping many things in the bud with its "yes, but...". It has probably managed to do this many times, especially with people on the spiritual path. For this reason, the ego looks out into the world with a corresponding sense of self-confidence and is quite confident about being able to get through with its usual tricks this time as well. This attitude is, of course, very understandable. The ego not only has a lot to lose, but in the long run, in fact everything. The best idea is to keep an eye on it at all times and to always watch out for its little games. In this way, they become more and more transparent over time.

Practical Exercise

Ask someone close to you, who you are connected to, without the additional demands of being in a relationship together; in other words, preferably someone from your circle of best friends, your brothers and sisters or parents, for an honest shadow conversation. Give this person express permission to be maximally direct and honest and make sure you take responsibility for their openness yourself. Release them from any potential negative consequences. Let this person tell you what he or she likes most and what he or she likes least about you. It is important that you do not interrupt your conversation partner, but instead listen silently and attentively, and that you also record what has been said. In this way, you will already gather essential points for your positive shadow list of those qualities that you want to realize, as well as for your negative list of those qualities that you will have to face without really wanting to. Both aspects are part of the shadow, as will be seen.

Those who already know what to expect on the part of the ego will not fall for its tricks as easily.

Just as important to us as our friends and loved ones on this path of confrontation with the shadow are our opponents, enemies and strangers, because they help us with their unconscious honesty. Involuntarily, they reflect back the shadows hidden within us that we are trying to project onto them instead. By simply being exactly as they and by displaying the shadow aspects that we recognize in them and reject, they remind us of our task. They create a connection to our shadow that is comparable to the role played by the golden ball for the princess in the fairy tale *The Frog Prince* (more on this in the chapter "Fairy tales and myths as signposts" starting on page 123). In this way, every enemy and opponent actually also passes the ball to us; when it comes to shadow work. In effect, they play into our hands and provide the perfect setup for a goal that is impossible to miss.

People in the East, for example in India, find all of this a little easier to deal with than we do in Western society. In principle, they are better at seeing through the ego's game, and our world of polarities is regarded from the outset as a form of deception or an illusion. This world, which they call Maya, is seen as being constructed from the two great deceivers: space and time. It is the ancestral home of ego and shadow. But even this better starting point does not prevent many people from Hindu and Buddhist cultures from also becoming victims of their own shadows in today's society.

In general, Fate works actively to support us, and with the help of the Law of Resonance, constantly draws us into contact with topics that are now due for integration. In this way, we become magnets for all external correspondences (resonances) with our unresolved problems and topics. They are presented to us on the stage of the outside world almost as though they are being served to us on a silver platter. The whole purpose of destiny seems to be to finally lead us to perfection, even if the process is often painful. That is why Fate constantly creates relationships with people and situations that reflect forgotten and repressed aspects and qualities of our being. And most of the time, these have to do with our shadow, our main task and challenge in life. Consequently, this means that if we suppress our own selfishness, we will constantly run into selfish people. Or vice versa, if we often run into selfish people who bother us, we can assume that we are selfish ourselves without having been prepared to admit it enough so far. In everyday life, we often then try to dodge into the opposite pole as an evasion tactic and to display as little selfishness as possible. As a result, this aspect disappears into the shadow realm. For this reason, those who, with the help of their clever ego, are constantly trying to prove how truly unselfish they are have every reason to be sceptical of such forms of "proof". Demonstrative altruism and deliberately-displayed charity are more an indication of an ego shadow than of what is supposedly being demonstrated.

If I feel like I am surrounded by arrogant people, I must be arrogant myself without being sufficiently aware of it. If this were not the case, arrogant people could neither trigger anything in me, nor would I attract so many of them around me. Or: If stupidity upsets me and I am constantly confronted by it, I must have no contact to a part of me that is (or has remained) stupid. Otherwise, it would not be an issue in my environment. On the other hand, however, it can also point towards polarity if I have placed too much emphasis on intellectual aspects in my life.

Without exception, whether we have something to do with a particular topic is revealed by our emotional reaction. Whatever moves, upsets or bothers us emotionally betrays our involvement, and we can be relatively certain that we are actually dealing with a problem of our own which has been projected outwards. If, on the other hand, something does not bother us emotionally, and we instead merely take note of it in a calm manner, it is no longer necessary to assume either projection or self-involvement. Not every piece of information we take in affects us. But as long as we necessarily have to do the opposite, for example, or are very proud of doing so, we are not yet free of the topic involved. We find this, for instance, when people stress

Shadow diary

When, where, how and in what way do I try to prove that I definitely do not have a certain characteristic, or that I definitely do not correspond to a certain pattern?

Look at situations in your life where you do the exact opposite in order to prove that you have nothing in common with the original characteristic. For example, have you ever been demonstratively generous so as not to appear as stingy as you really are? Or have you ever been demonstratively hardworking in order not to appear as lazy as you actually are?

that they are definitely nothing like their parents. A good sign that freedom from a particular topic has been achieved is if one can shed light on it without getting emotional and can freely consider its various different sides.

The opportunity to gain a further degree of inner clarity often comes in surprising ways. An example of this is an experience that enabled me to learn more about my shadow: Many years ago, I had found a beautiful island in the Philippine archipelago that came very close to my idea of paradise on Earth. It was a very small island with just a few islanders, who lived a simple life and constantly gave us the opportunity to do good without any effort and even—a must for young doctors—to save lives. The islanders only lived on one half of the island. The other side of the island was deserted and more idyllic than travel catalogues showed it to be: a wide, snow-white coral beach of the finest sand, the sea a veritable dream for divers and full of fish that did not seem to be afraid of people. I built several beautiful bamboo houses on a cliff behind the beach, whose location and view couldn't have been more picturesque. It was here that I wanted to retreat and meditate and enjoy an idyllic life. Later Thorwald Dethlefsen joined me, and we planned to write books and design seminars—in paradise, so to speak.

Nevertheless, we soon realized that we were able to be more creative everywhere else in the world than here of all places. At first, we blamed this on external superficialities, like the lack of refrigerators and air conditioners. However, even after we had worked through the list of trivialities, we remained relatively unproductive, and our book *The Healing Power of Illness* failed to progress. It took a while for us to realize how deeply we were resonating with paradise, and to understand that, on this dream island, there was neither any reason, nor any driving motivation to deal with shadow issues, such as illness. Significantly, this realization did not reduce our interest in disease patterns in the long run, but instead our desire for the island paradise. Our shadow still wanted a showdown with us, and we wanted to undertake this in the form of thinking, writing and talking—in projection, so to speak—rather than having to suffer it physically in our own bodies.

When once again we came back to the island some time later, there was finally something to do and to criticize. Our paradise was tarnished, and from afar, we were horrified by the presence of a fence. A doctor that we were friends with had erected the fence around the houses. As the only fence on the island, it was an eyesore for us and a thorn in our side. The friend refused to tear down the fence, which served to protect his daughter from dogs and pigs. But the question remained: Why could a simple fence drive us up the wall?

With the help of mutual psychotherapy, the problem quickly became clear in my inner world of images: Coming from Germany, a tightly-restricted world full of fences and walls, and at that time, still the home of the Wall par excellence, I did not want to be reminded, here of all places, of the limitations that we had brought with us. As such, the small fence that in turn fenced off and confined a smaller piece of our paradise became threatening. In the inner world of images, the connection became clear to me when I was confronted with the question of which inner fence of my own this external fence reminded me of. The fence appeared immediately—and it was not smaller and less significant, as I had suspected, since I had considered myself to be broad-minded and open with respect to integration. No, my fence was huge; it surrounded the whole island, "my island", and it reached so far into the sea that it was invisible from the beach. I had chosen this island because everything ran according to my ideas: the pleasantly-quiet life of the locals, the wonderful flora, in fact, every facet of nature on the island, and the islanders who lived in harmony with it. I didn't have to put up a fence because of the island's character. The only disturbance was something that I had brought in myself in the form of my friend and his fence, which then reminded me of my own much larger one. In the rest of the session, the multifaceted inner fences, with which I separated myself and secured my ego, were also effortlessly brought to the surface by Thorwald. After that, I could look at the fence around the huts and also its builder in a different way.

This example may make clear just how close we often are to finding the solution to a (shadow) problem. So how do we proceed in concrete terms?

- The first step is to identify the shadow. In this regard, we can never run out of material, because everything that we dislike or resist is basically a possible source of shadow. Shadow is hidden in everything that we disagree with or that we cannot identify ourselves with. This can be just as much our annoyance at our neighbour, as the indignation we feel about a major injustice in social or political life. Why, for example, did the wall that divided Germany upset the majority of people in the West so much, even though most of them were not directly affected? The political leaders of the German Democratic Republic, who were a constant target of projection from the people in the West, chose to forcibly set themselves and their citizens apart from us in this way. If this wall bothered us, was it because it reminded us of our own inner walls? If we felt particularly provoked by the fact that the Socialist Unity Party of East Germany had locked away its own people so that they would not attempt to flee, then we should also apply this aspect to our own inner world. Is it possible that we, too, are locking away something inside of us? Is it perhaps true that we build inner walls, so that we do not fall apart as a personality because our individual character traits do not bond together easily to form a harmonious whole? Do we need a high wall to lock away the inner shadow realm from a life in freedom?

And why did we get so worked up about the apartheid regime of the South African Boers? After all, South Africa is far away and most of us had no first-hand experience of it. But it reminded us of our own inner apartheid, of our detachment and separation from our dark side. In the same way that the white Boers excluded and locked away the blacks, and hence the majority of the population, in Townships, we lock away our own dark sides, fence them in and do not let them take part in our life.

Is it possible that we are so strongly opposed to the keeping of chickens in battery cages because this reminds us of the correspondingly cooped-up way of life of many people in modern cities? Some may be directly affected themselves; others may have a guilty conscience because they can afford a better lifestyle than the majority.

- The second step leads to the question: What does this have to do with me? More precisely, it is no longer about whether it has to do with me, but only in what way I am affected by it. At any rate, it either happened to me or at least bothered me. Everything, no matter how disagreeable, always has to do with me, because I experience it and react emotionally to it. Otherwise I could neither experience it, nor could it trigger emotions in me.
- In the subsequent third step, we have to find out on which level we are representing and living the corresponding topic. Even in cases, where the shadow aspect is extremely unpleasant and what has happened to me may be incredibly unfair, a coherent connection can be found. On the one hand, this puts our honesty regarding ourselves to a tough test, and on the other hand, calls for great creativity. In this respect, there is no shame in getting professional help in the form of shadow therapy.
- The fourth step is a ritual of forgiveness. In the truest sense of the word, it is necessary to forgive precisely the darkest shadow aspects of oneself. To this end, we should make clear to ourselves what this shadow has brought us/taught us; what it has confronted us with. In this way, it is easier to recognize with one's heart, one's whole being, how necessary this aspect was for our development and our progress. For the ritual of forgiveness, it is helpful to relax and allow the particular shadow aspect in question to appear before one's inner eye—either symbolically or as a concrete person or situation. While still in this relaxed state, send your thanks to the circumstance or that person

on the inner-imagery level of the soul for providing the impetus for development. Afterwards, it is easy to consciously admit to oneself: I am as I am and am allowed to be as I am and can now freely make use of the energy involved with this shadow aspect as I choose.

This self-forgiveness requires the consciousness of a ritual; just thinking about it is not enough. It is important to sit or lie down in a special place, and to take the time to be in a special state of consciousness. And while we devote ourselves inwardly to the moment of self-forgiveness, we should also feel it deeply in our heart: "I am allowed to be exactly as I am. Otherwise, Creation/God would not have made me in this way".

In addition, there is a further gift in this ritual: "Forgiveness," said Nelson Mandela, "eliminates fear". And of all people, he definitely should know the truth of that, since, even while he was still alive, he had already gone down in history as the champion of forgiveness. He essentially managed to reconcile his internally-torn land, which had been split into two halves and was at the mercy of the respective shadow aspects of the two opposing sides, through the power of forgiveness. Two ideal journeys on the subject can be found on the CD *The Healing Power of Forgiveness**.

- The fifth step is to devote attention to the corresponding shadow aspect. Nevertheless, we are used to doing the exact opposite, and throughout the years, we have trained the reverse tendency, namely to push away everything that is unpleasant as best we can, or at the very least, to ignore it. A symptom, such as a cut that has been unintentionally inflicted on me, by a stranger (enemy) or perhaps even by myself can perhaps serve as an illustrative example. Regardless of how I ended up with it, I will regard this symptom as hostile like any other. I don't want it. Make it go away. In this case, as with all other symptoms, it will do that, and will do so far more quickly, the more I tend to it and treat it in a caring way. Even though I am not happy about it, I will tend to the wound and take care to cleanse it properly. If I can manage to cleanse it in depth, I can then close it (or let it be closed) and thus promote its healing. Alternatively, I can keep the wound open and allow it to bleed freely, thus enabling the blood to remove the dirt. This also has the added advantage of exposing it to air to promote healing and to prevent complications, such as tetanus. I can also treat the aura above this part of the body with Reiki or with other energy-related exercises, such as simply offering to kiss it better, which almost all mothers instinctively do anyway, all the way up to Deeksha, the rediscovered ancient form of the Hindu blessing.

Turning our attention towards something that we do not actually want to have is a matter of course in the case of the cut. However, it is also the decisive step in other cases, and shows how medicine in the sense of *Disease as a Symbol* can be transferred to many situations. Suppressing or ignoring symptoms does not help. People with chronic clinical illness patterns often live with their symptoms in solid enmity in a very confined space for many decades, without experiencing any improvement. Affection and reconciliation, on the other hand, do help.

An example such as that offered by depression may show in depth how much sense there is in every symptom, regardless of whether we see through its origin or not. If we can put aside our judgement for a moment, it can be recognized almost as a work of art. Depressive people have a lot of time on their hands due to their frequent sleep disorders. They are forced to use most of it worrying more or less continuously about the pointlessness of their lives and torturing themselves with thoughts of suicide. In this way, they deal, albeit on an unresolved level, with their central problems and the task that is entailed in them: mortality, finiteness, death. Fortunately, due to their lack of drive, they usually remain completely blocked in the phase of deep depression and are thus unable to put their suicidal thoughts into practice. That particular danger exists only once they start to re-surface from the depths of the dark night of the soul. In the meantime, the symptoms of depression force them to be entirely present in the here and now and give them—in a relatively-protected state—all the time in the world to deal with their problems. In doing so, the brain defaults to an earlier mode of operation that is just sufficient to allow the pending emergency program to be carried out. If we turn our attention to a symptom, disease or any other shadow aspect, these phenomena can teach us what we are lacking. The cut shows us in a plain and simple way that we have cut ourselves off from a part of ourselves—in the sense of self-delusion—and that we need to stitch up the two sides of this renewed split in the short or medium term in order to achieve healing. Depression shows us that the topic of mortality and death is sorely lacking in our life and that life in the here and now is finally claiming its rightful place. In a similar way, all symptoms and shadow aspects bring us back to ourselves when we respect and respond to them.

Nevertheless, as soon as people in our society get into difficulties or have problems they need to solve, most of them prefer to rely on their rational mind first and foremost. Admittedly, it does its best, but it is also full of prejudices. Despite this, within the context of shadow work, it can be of great help in finding the topic in general and in finding the respective level of concern.

For the concrete shadow work of reconciliation, the attitude of "not knowing", as practised by Buddhists, is ideal. This is free of prejudice, or characterized by Uppekha—a state of equanimity or positive indifference towards the observation of shadow events, as though we are perceiving something in which we are more a witness than a participant.

For shadow work, it is a good idea to tone down the influence of our intellect a little bit since we are constantly using it to twist and contort things. This is possible, for example, when we write things down—instead of just thinking or saying them—because the intellect is slowed down in its pace when writing. Moreover, as soon as we start to not only spontaneously and intuitively express the first thought, but also to write it down, this undermines the rationalization methods of the intellect even more. If

Practical Exercise

Sit or lie down in as relaxed a state as possible, and simply wait and see which moods and emotions make themselves felt without any action on your part. Imagine that you are a guest in the house that is your own body, and just sit back and observe the guests who enter and make themselves at home for a certain period of time. Each of these guests has a message for you as the host or hostess with regard to your emotional state. No guest could enter if you did not have any resonance with them, and typically, it will be the shadow topics that attract uninvited and unpleasant guests. If you dedicate a quarter of an hour every morning to this Uppekha (equanimity) exercise, over time, you will project your own negative vibes less and less onto the people around you.

this writing process can mimic the perspective of a child, who does not yet care about style and grammar, but simply wants to get its feelings off its chest, all the better. Incidentally, this is also the ideal stance to take when writing the shadow diary. Naturally, this means that structure and order in the outer world will suffer somewhat, but our involvement in the inner world will be increased, which is the main issue.

Even more can be expressed in painting. Directly after each shadow therapy session at the *Heilkundezentrum*—our healing centre in Bavaria, Germany—we not only ask the patients to write down their experiences, but also encourage them to represent them in paint so that they can examine these in even greater depth. Thoughts must be "ex-pressed" in the truest sense of the word, namely of "pressing out something" into a form, which can then be let out into the world. After painting or writing, the next logical step would be to publish everything openly, just I have done to a certain extent in this book by hinting at some of my own shadow aspects. It would, of course, be the most far-reaching possibility of expression, but typically remains just a theory that is rarely put into practice. Nevertheless, doing so would show how unconditionally one stands by one's own dark sides. What is quite manageable, however, is to put what has become clear to you about the shadow in words and then tell this to someone who is important to you in your own life.

How masks develop

The development of our personality, or in other words, the formation of our conscious self, is founded on judgements. The persona develops as a mask and facade. This process can be illustrated as follows:

We are sent into life with a comprehensive set of basic mental and emotional configurations. Even as infants, we then already experience which of our predispositions go down well with our parents, and especially, with our mother. These characteristics become strongly reinforced, while others that do not win favor may not be allowed to develop since they are not tolerated so gladly. As a result, these slip out of sight and ultimately into the shadows.

If toddlers experience how aggressive attempts to assert their own will repeatedly trigger strong disapproval on the part of their parents or even lead to punishment, they will unconsciously devalue such attempts and eventually give up. On the other hand, lovable obedience will be assigned a higher value and strengthened. In this way, we constantly decide between opposite poles right from the very beginning and develop what we call "personality" in the course of what parents call "child-raising". Over time, children learn by means of the mirror of their environment to replace unpopular traits with their respective opposites. For this process, it makes no difference whether they are beaten, scolded or indirectly belittled for these undesirable qualities, for example, by being warned: "The good Lord is sad when you do that!" In contrast, parents who encourage their child to stand up for itself, to go into bat for its interests, and if necessary, to fight for these will naturally cause less shadow formation in the child on the one hand and encourage more self-confidence on the other.

At this point, it is important to once again be very clear about the fact that the things that we have rejected and now no longer show still remain present, and by no means, cease to exist; they have simply sunk deep into the shadows. All we can ever manage to do is merely to hide them. The shadow realm thus becomes the hiding place for everything that is unloved and not tolerated by our parents, our environment and finally even by ourselves. Science knows about the principle of energy conservation, according to which energy can never actually disappear, but instead can only be transformed into other manifestations. When water freezes to ice or evaporates to gas, none of its molecules disappears. The same applies to mental-emotional energies: Shifting mental energy from consciousness into the unconscious or from the ego into the realm of the shadow is easy; it is the way back from the realm of the shadow into consciousness that is the problem—and the main concern of this book. Different forms of energy never disappear; it is merely our level of consciousness of them that changes.

As development progresses, the spectrum of characteristics that children show becomes smaller and smaller. What has survived judgement by the parents is next exposed to the judgement of the extended family and further judged by this larger circle in turn. In the process, quite a few things are once again sorted out and pushed into the shadows. Following on from

Meditation

Read Meditations 1 & 7 aloud to yourself and then allow yourself sufficient time afterwards for the meditation to come to a harmonious close.

Following this, confide your experiences to your shadow diary.

this, the friends in our age group, our so-called "peer group, make their own judgmental selection of what is "in" and "out". Naturally, the "in" and "out" lists in youth magazines play the same tune. What is "out" has to go—the last resort is always the shadow realm.

In this way, throughout our lifetime, we put all of the spiritual-emotional gifts that we brought with us and later also our acquired abilities into the shop display window of our lives. What is not well received and not well accepted by the general public disappears again first to the back shelves, then under the counter and finally into the shadow realm. In this way, we decide via trial and error what to keep in our persona(lity) and what we shove down into the shadows. It is therefore ultimately our environment that decides what is acceptable and may remain and what must instead remain in our shadow (sack). By the time we have put kindergarten, school, university studies, an apprenticeship or other vocational training behind us, the offer in our display window has already been greatly reduced. At this point, it may also have already become clear how immensely important the quality of our family home and other educational institutions is.

The more we sort out and reject in childhood and our youth, the less we have to offer in adolescence (in our display window)—and the larger our shadow arsenal becomes. Unfortunately, it is not always the best and most valuable traits, nor the most useful or most meaningful aspects that remain, but rather whatever best conforms to and suits the majority. It is via this mechanism that the silent majority, or as it often referred to, the "mainstream" ensures its continuing stability. With each job and relationship that we leave in our wake, we have less and less to (put on) offer in the display window of our lives.

Supply and demand also regulate each other at this level. What is not bought is removed after a while and lands on the bottom shelf. Over time, this leads to a larger collection of poor selling items, which we call shadow. Unfortunately, the characteristics and traits that have been ignored by those around us are also dumped. And in the end, we, our persona(lity), are really only what always went down well.

Only if we learned in our parental home to defend our character(istics), or even better, if we were allowed to experience being loved unconditionally, can we preserve more of our riches. If not, our personality will have shrunk to a small collection of qualities that are generally-accepted on the path of life. All of the rest is shadow, and the stricter and narrower our surroundings were, the greater the shadow realm, but at the same time, the more valuable this shadow realm will be if we are successful in bringing these deeply-buried treasures back into our life.

This phenomenon of a continual increase in shadow over time can be found everywhere. If we look at Christianity today in the wake of the Inquisition, the Crusades and the current catastrophe of child abuse, we are presented with an image of shadow. If we had made our observation in the first century after Christ, the bright sides would have dominated. The same is probably true of our own relationship. In the first year, a bright picture of radiant love was presented; but after ten years, the shadow aspects often predominate. Where there is so much shadow, there must also have been so much light. Eventually, all of the shadows come out. This is something we can be entirely certain of; it is always only a question of time.

What is particularly unfortunate about all of this, is that, in the way described above, things slip into the shadows that later on most certainly would have found favour with others. By that point, however, they had already been sorted out and rejected. Unfortunately, for most people, the following motto applies: once in the shadow, always in the shadow. A person who is constantly in and out of relationships will indeed gain experience, but in each one—usually without noticing it—will also sacrifice certain topics and characteristics. Some of these might have gone down really well in later relationships, but now they are no longer even on offer, and thus didn't get a second chance.

This explains why, with increasing age, many people actually reduce their repertoire instead of growing mentally and spiritually. The most disturbing aspect about this in my eyes is how many people get so used to their reduced self-image that, in the end, they not only accept, but even like it in its reduced form. They now no longer take the offensive in life, having been ground down smooth, but they are quick to take offence at everything that differs from them and that is still vibrant and full of life. They themselves no longer provide any impetus or stimulus for growth. Having already "died" early, they are often buried only late. They no longer feel their enormous resistance to life, because they have almost completely excluded whatever is still full of life. What they refer to as their "life" hardly deserves this name anymore and has more to do with the demands of their respective society than with them personally, or with their individuality. That is why many older people seem so reduced in their possibilities; their personality is limited and their shadow enormous. Their remaining life opportunities are only minimal if they do not integrate the shadow with its great wealth. Those who have understood the underlying pattern behind cancer in the sense of my book *Disease as a Language of the Soul* should easily recognize at this point why, in keeping with the content of this disease pattern, its incidence also increases with age. Growth that is no longer lived on levels of consciousness increasingly sinks into the shadows or into the body.

The few things that remain, because they fit into the narrow world view of the respective society, often seem boring. Far more exciting would be the things that make up the shadow, and above all, the stories that are intertwined with it. The heroine in the cult film *Harold and Maude* is a splendid example of a person who has not surrendered to the dictates of society with its compulsion to hide behind masks. Maude beautifully portrays the archetype of the crazy old woman. Few things require as much courage as being eccentric (literally: "off centre") and leaving the safety of the herd. Maude has managed this despite surviving the horrors of a concentration camp. External authorities, such as police officers, traffic rules and driving licence regulations are simply no longer important in her life when compared to such essential aspects as feelings, emotions, sensual impressions and questions about the deeper meaning of life. She looks at every moment with the astonished wonderment of a child and thus seems to have managed to "become like the children". Even death has lost all terror for her. From the point of view of society, the old Maude is acting crazy, but she does so in an enchanting and fascinating way. And in her own eccentric manner, she is reconciled with the topics of age and death. What becomes clear here is that there is great wealth to be found in the shadow—old jewels that are authentic, original and sparkle with vitality.

It is *the* major decision that we make in life whether we allow ourselves to stay limited to the life that is left over, so to speak, after all of the sorting out and rejection processes have taken place, or instead begin to heal the past and integrate the shadow. A wise old saying among therapists is that: "it is never too late to have

Shadow diary

Part 1: What would be the worst that my mother, my father could say about me? What is the worst my partner could say about me? What is the worst my child(ren) could say about me? What would be the worst thing my most important teacher could say about me? What is the worst that my most important trainer or coach could say against me? What would be the worst thing that could be written about me in the (local) newspaper? What could be reported about me on radio and television in the worst case scenario?

Be aware that everything you have written down in response to these questions is also true and part of the shadow. What we are afraid of comes into our lives in one form or another. Once again, it is merely a question of levels and does not have to happen as we fear. Nevertheless, the corresponding energy will surface in whatever context is appropriate to our lives.

Part 2: Repeat the above game and replace the word "worst" with "nicest" to find the positive light shadow of your life: What would be the nicest thing my mother, my father, my partner, my child(ren), my most important teacher, my most important trainer or coach could say about me? What would be the best thing that could be reported about me in the (local) newspaper, or on radio and television?

If you find yourself wanting to skip this pleasant part because it is too much for you right now, you can also quickly interpret the shadow straightaway.

a happy childhood." If we ignore this adage, the shadow becomes more and more powerful and eventually suffocates the best parts of us. Nevertheless, it is hard to say for sure which option is better: is it preferable for the shadow to become overpowering in the sense of a psychosis and take over complete control in life, but at least make its existence felt? Or are we better off if the shadow becomes overpowering in the bourgeois sense, burying everything that is spontaneous, creative, original and spiritual under it and leaving only robot-like functioning. In psychosis, the shadow is able to live out in the open, whereas in the zombie-like existence of the remote-controlled robot, it lives in hiding—and the danger of uncontrolled outbreaks constantly grows. Here, the trained eyes of a therapist are necessary to be able to discover the shadow that is lurking behind the rigidities, blocks, symptoms and slip-ups and then lure it out.

If we start tracking down our own shadow themes, our family of origin is a good initial orientation guide. Whatever does not fit into their quite clearly-defined frame inevitably falls into the shadow. As a result, (great-)grandparents and other ancestors play an important role alongside parents.

A look at our parents shows us most clearly what was allowed to stay and what consequently has now remained. When

Film Meditation

Watch the film Harold and Maude in a state of meditative relaxation. Pay particularly conscious attention to the multifaceted masked ball in Harold's family and enjoy the authenticity of Maude's shadow realm. Afterwards, as the music of the closing credits fades, allow yourself to enter your own world of touching child-like authenticity and then also your own masked ball. Record your impressions and thoughts in your shadow diary.

it comes to topics that have been granted an important place in their soul, they can and could easily accept these in us as well. Whatever they did not tolerate in themselves, however, probably was also not allowed to remain in our shop window and therefore ended up in the shadow. For this reason, it is important to comb through

our family of origin with regard to such values. The easiest way to do this is on the level of inner imagery in the sense of a guided meditation.

The analysis of our parents and their values and expectations, which have left their imprint on our original family, will yield the shadow that has been repressed the longest on the shadow side. Topics that already had no place with parents and grandparents and that have been poorly tolerated in our culture in general form extremely deep shadows that stretch all the way back to the collective shadow. Sexuality, for example, could be buried in the deep shadow layers because it is poorly regarded in Christian culture. Aggression, on the other hand, is usually less deeply repressed, since it is much more accepted. Excessive violence on television hardly upsets anyone, but comparable sex orgies are in contrast completely unthinkable.

Be aware that parents act as developmental assistants for Fate and should therefore not be abused as the projection surface for the creation of new shadow. As a rule, your parents have done everything they could to get you to this point in your

Meditation

Read Meditations 1 & 8 aloud to yourself and then allow yourself sufficient time afterwards for the meditation to come to a harmonious close.

Following this, confide your experiences to your shadow diary.

life. Now it is all about focussing on you yourself and leaving the projections behind. As our lives progress, the pressure (of our upbringing) on what is offered in the display window of our lives decreases significantly. The older we get, the less we are told what to do and the more we can be as we want. While the initial pressure to adapt in childhood is strong, it eases off palpably later and is barely relevant by mid-life. These different periods can be clarified with the help of meditation exercises.

Forces of attraction—the people in my life

The stricter and more restrictive a child's environment was, the fewer of its sides it will have been able to accept, and the more the few remaining aspects of its persona(lity) will later be reinforced and emphasized. The child's ego will become narrow, rigid and entrenched and its shadow large and extensive.

In contrast, the more understanding, open, constructive and supportive the environment was, the more everything that belongs to the character(istics) of the child will have been accepted. Correspondingly, the ego will have become less rigid and the shadow will not have developed on such a massive scale. Consciousness, on the other hand, widens and expands to the extent that the shadow remains more modest.

A person with a massive ego will radiate something superimposed, rushed, strained and artificial. With a less entrenched, open and transparent ego, on the other hand, we experience the person concerned as authentic and genuine; they seem closer to their sense of self and to self-actualization in general. This also means that more shadow has already been integrated. In this respect, an open, liberal starting point is a great gift for every child and offers the chance to confront the shadow more easily and more successfully. Admittedly, for people who initially experienced only restriction and constraint, the need for shadow confrontation is particularly great, but since the shadow is usually formidable, there is less chance that the person concerned will dare to approach it. In this case, the reward would be particularly substantial. Nevertheless, the challenge for a more entrenched and tighty-constrained ego is also particularly tough, which results in a typical vicious circle.

What is able to emerge from deep within us in terms of shadow and can thus be brought to light is revealed through correspondingly appropriate people and situations. In accordance with the Law of Resonance, we constantly attract certain types of people, who help us by acting as mirrors—without wanting to or even suspecting it. This applies to parents, as well as to partners and bosses. Fate can be totally relied upon in this respect. If we have truly integrated a shadow topic, these people vanish from our lives. They either become less important for us or they stop showing us the troubling behaviour. Alternatively, we suddenly find ourselves easily able to part company with them, and in any case, we no longer allow ourselves to be provoked by them.

The more shadow topics we integrate of our own free will, the fewer mirrors we need to make ourselves aware of them, and the calmer and more relaxed our surrounding environment becomes. The more shadow we have integrated and that is allowed to exist out in the open, the more the people around us will mirror this back to us. In contrast, what we condemn in others shows what we are still refusing to own up to in ourselves; it has not been integrated and therefore remains part of our shadow. It cannot be repeated often enough: Whoever or whatever goes against the grain for us is part of our shadow. Whoever or whatever we find offensive and that therefore puts us on the offensive is also part of our shadow.

Shadow diary

What kind of people do I attract nowadays, and what was it like in the past? What does that say about my shadow? Which topics do the people around me mirror for me with respect to my development and my shadow?

In addition, consider the main characteristics of your current best friend and "dearest" enemy. Record your thoughts and findings in your shadow diary.

We all encounter the correspondingly appropriate people and situations on our path through life. This can mean, for example, that the sicker the doctor is himself, the more seriously ill his patients will be. The more therapists manage to unravel and solve their own entanglements and problems, the healthier and better developed will be the people who are able to seek out and accept their help. The more we accept about ourselves, the more perfectly rounded will be those who come into our lives and share it with us.

Romantic relationships work via projection both in good times and in bad. Behind the positive qualities that I see in my partner right at the very beginning in the early phase of being madly in love are my own positive development wishes that I project onto him or her. I would love to be as charming, fascinating, beautiful, intelligent, successful, eloquent, kind, musical, down-to-earth or unconventional, and at the very least, lovable. If I actually tried to develop these qualities within myself from the very beginning, the relationship could be the stimulus for my own development right from the start. This phase of the relationship clearly illustrates the Law of Resonance. We resonate together in harmony, because we consciously allow ourselves to be open to one another and we are enthusiastic about our own positive projections. The relationship energy at this point is characterized by positive or light shadow.

The next phase is governed by the Law of Polarity. At this point, everything starts to become more difficult. My partner now begins to mirror my own dark shadow aspects, which I certainly do not want to admit to, let alone accept, and which I am not even able to recognize. Admittedly, I actually carry them within me—and to that extent I am also in resonance with them—but they seem completely foreign to me and even seem to reflect the total opposite of me. In this way, I now experience how my partner is showing me my opposite pole. In him or her, I see all the more clearly what I do not like and do not want to recognize in myself, and I may even start to fight this in him or her—and thus in effect, in the projection itself. In actual fact, the partner doesn't do anything. I am the one who pushes my own unlived/unloved aspects onto him or her, and who having seen these, then begins attacking them in him or her. Typically, this dynamic eventually ruins the relationship if we do not finally realize that we can only ever judge and abuse, insult and fight ourselves. Our dark shadow, which is easily recognized in our projection of it onto our partner, but hardly ever in ourselves, develops more and more explosive potential and often causes the relationship to fail in the end.

Relationships are therefore an ideal training ground for shadow work. We could learn to take back both our positive, light shadow aspects, and in the long term, also the negative, dark ones. In the end, it is all about learning to love our enemies, but also of course our friends, and above all, ourselves.

With friends and enemies, we also have a kind of relationship. Both types of relationship benefit equally from a peculiar effect that keeps both friendships or enmity going. Once we have sorted someone into a pigeonhole and cloaked them with some kind of projection, we tend to stick with it. With friends this is referred to as the "halo effect". No matter what they do—we attach our own positive projections to them. Once we have grown fond of them, we give them carte blanche and they can get away with anything. In contrast, no matter what our enemies do, they will never manage to get out of the dark corner we have put them in. Once someone has become enemy number one in a group or department, family or company, they will have a hard time shaking this label.

In many modern industrialized countries, the divorce rate has risen from eighteen to almost eighty percent within the last fifty years. This development in the domain of relationships shows how little work is being done on the shadow. Most people in relationships fight in vain, but nonetheless with great devotion, against the mirror, i.e. against the behaviour of the partner, and in doing so, leave the shadow untouched. The only sensible way out is for us to once again own up to the unconscious aspects of ourselves in terms of shadow therapy. We then no longer have to shift the blame to our partner, but can, on the contrary, turn these into gold for our own path or our joint path together. That is the actual task in relationships and love. Nothing else can help us as effectively in our dealings with the shadow. When we learn to love what is, nothing can befall us except our final call back to the kingdom of heaven. Erich Fried sees it in this way as well and expresses the goal of the path in his poem "Was es ist" (What it is):

It is nonsense
says reason
It is what it is
says love

It is calamity
says calculation
It is nothing but pain
says fear

It is hopeless
says insight
It is what it is
says love

It is ludicrous
says pride
It is foolish
says caution
It is impossible
says experience
It is what it is
says love

In contrast, in line with polarity, Heinrich Heine puts it as follows:

The angels call it heavenly joy
The devils call it hellish suffering
Humans call it love.

Shadow games and personality

As we already know, our persona is the mask that only reveals what our Self considers to be acceptable and that holds back everything that belongs to the shadow. Only sometimes, something manages to slip past the mask, a small faux pas occurs, a "misstep" that allows shadow material to escape. This is what leads to slips of the tongue, oversights, slip-ups, blunders and trip-ups. We could regard all of these as little tricks that are played on us by our shadow in order to smuggle itself into everyday life.

Suggestions for learning more about the shadow and relationships

The audio program Relationships* offers two guided meditations on the topic of shadow in relationships, which can then help to transform it. The film classic *Who's Afraid of Virginia Woolf?*, starring Elizabeth Taylor and Richard Burton in the leading roles, also portrays the dark shadow in relationships in an unsurpassed way. The film *The War of the Roses*" with Kathleen Turner and Michael Douglas depicts a similarly exhausting marriage duel and the typical change from light into shadow in a relationship. For examples of the light shadow in relationships, there are countless love films. Ingmar Bergman's *Scenes from a Marriage* is particularly successful in showing the whole drama, but also newer ones, such as *As Good as it Gets* with Jack Nicholson und Helen Hunt. Each of these films offers us the opportunity to take the magic words "The End" as the beginning of our own story, to close our eyes and to look at our own shadows. Anyone who is not currently in a relationship probably has this as a shadow topic. However, he or she can also experience the relevant learning steps through friends, colleagues, bosses and neighbours—albeit usually with less intensity. Regardless of which of the suggestions offered here for your shadow work you choose, don't forget to note your insights and thoughts in your shadow diary.

In a similar way, disease symptoms develop from inner shadow pressure, but have a more lasting effect and far more energy behind them. They are more or less massive representations of the shadow, which the latter uses to lodge itself firmly in our conscious life. Acute symptoms are more like the sudden slip-ups; in the case of chronic symptoms, however, the shadow energy has already managed to enforce its influence in a lasting and sustainable way. That is why we want to get rid of the symptoms and what they signify and symbolize as quickly as possible.

An army of therapists who are unacquainted with the shadow uses allopathic approaches and psychological and social repression to join forces against the Unconscious. In the long run, though, the shadow has more leverage, as it occupies the centre of power, namely the core of our being. In contrast, the mask of the person(a) is comparably superficial, and any repression measures also only work on the surface.

If, for example, a person(a) presents a fun-loving exterior, while a sad being hides within the depths, as with the great depressive clowns throughout circus history, in the worst case scenario, the amusement will seem more and more superimposed over the years. The jokes will become cruder and the laughter will become louder in an attempt to withstand the growing shadow pressure. In contrast, truly great clowns find access to their dark side, and as a result, their humour becomes subtle and profound, and the laughter that they trigger then acts as a release, reminding the people in the audience of their own depths.

The full repertoire in the masked ball of life is tremendous. Not just the number of costumes and roles, but also the many different types of balls that they are used at. Behind cool designer stubble, it is not uncommon to find insecure guys who are lacking confidence in their masculinity. They go to great lengths with special razors to act out a role on the surface that they are not (yet) up to playing in the depths. But what a guy in his twenties might get away with, already seems a bit overdone for a man in his late forties. Extremely relaxed, die-hard hippies don a colourful costume of non-conformism in order to hide their tension with regard to responsibility and their fear of structure and order behind an elaborately-staged, laid-back exterior.

An exaggerated sense of importance often enters into relationships with demonstrative beauty. For anyone who can see through the masks of our personality, it is carnival or Mardi Gras all year round, because modern society has made us into masters of disguise. Early in life, we develop masks in order to avoid hurting anyone, to satisfy as many people as possible, and above all, not to challenge our(S)elf. Calibrated for the path of least resistance, we definitely need a persona with a differentiated mask or facade. The larger and more anonymous a society or subculture is, and thus the greater the pressure to fit in, the more energy flows into the construction of the facade. For example, in the course of his shadow therapy, a priest discovered that he had a different face for baptisms, communions, confirmations, weddings and funerals, which he could call up on demand. This does not mean, however, that all masks of the persona are bad by definition; we should simply keep trying to be ourselves again and again and to only use the masks when necessary, instead of never taking them off, gradually stiffening behind them and thus eventually losing our (true) face.

The *Tao Te Ching* makes the dilemma clear in verse 76:

> People are born soft and supple;
> when they die, they are rigid and stiff.
> Plants are born flexible and tender;
> when they die, they are brittle and dry.
>
> Stiffness is thus a disciple of death;
> flexibility a disciple of life.
> An army that cannot yield
> will be defeated.
> A tree that cannot bend
> will crack in the wind.
>
> The hard and stiff will be broken.
> The soft and supple will prevail.

The persona, the mask we show to the world, becomes more and more necessary and increasingly rigid over the course of

> **Shadow diary**
>
> Where am I fixed and rigid in my body? Where hard and stubborn in my soul? Who could I ask for honest help with discovering insights? With whom could I really bear it if he or she helps me to see those shadows for which I am blinded (by myself)? Which friendship or relationship could withstand that?
>
> Please write down your answers and impressions in your shadow diary.

our life in order to continue hiding the shadow and to keep pace with the growing discrepancy with regard to the Self. The Self, or in other words, an ego that has integrated the shadow, is soft and supple. A person who has spent their whole life adapting to others and making the effort to please everyone will wind up totally stressed out in the end. This is because it is difficult to always have the various different masks at the ready and to be constantly changing them, while at the same time trying to withstand the inner shadow pressure. Christian or Buddhist hermits, for example, hardly need masks because during their monastic life they encounter no-one other than themselves in the solitude of their cell.

When it comes to the shadow, however, they also do not have it easy either. Without an external mirror, the shadow becomes invisible, yet it does not disappear. This explains the phenomenon that many Eastern gurus seemed enlightened in their home ashram and also felt enlightened. No sooner had they arrived in the West, however, with all its new temptations, than the unprocessed aspects, which had not yet been mirrored, came forward. Suddenly the "masters" seemed like con-artists. In effect, they had simply run aground on their own shadow.

Let us note then that, in the course of a person's life, the shadow takes on a stronger and clearer form, thereby exposing the person concerned to growing embarrassment. When our self-image and the image of us held by others bear little resemblance anymore, we feel like we have failed in life; the image of our existence crashing down around us forces itself upon us. The vast majority of people around us today grow up without any role models for inner spiritual development. For this reason, the persona is strongly preferred to the shadow and the Self. Most successful people have several masks and are highly adept at changing them at will. From here, it is only a small step to the sub-personalities and split-personalities of psychosynthesis, which we will come back to later. Those who, on the other hand, focus more on self-realization in the sense of C.G. Jung's individuation will place their shadow and shining light upon it as the central focal point of interest in their life.

In the different phases of life, the mask and the shadow will be assigned different weightings. In the first half of life, in line with the Christian mission of subjugating the Earth, the person(a) with its masks and facades may outweigh the shadow. This phase is all about being successful in the world, or in other words, externally. In the second half of life, however, when heading home and inner reflection regarding the soul are on the agenda, the shadow should receive the main attention, since it is now all about inner development and self-realization.

In any case, in both halves of life, different domains will require different levels of attention. In a relationship, shadow work and an inner connection could already be weighted more heavily to great advantage in the first half of life. In contrast, a modern profession may make it necessary to emphasize the persona beyond middle age. This will depend on the respective role. Not everyone in this society allows us to be genuine and forthright, open-minded and humane. Modern managers, bankers and C.E.O.s seem to have more difficulties in this respect; fasting doctors, course leaders and psychotherapists naturally have it much easier in this regard. The decision about whether to put spiritual development in first place or success in the world is something that each and every one of us can only make for ourselves. A reliable yardstick for this could be bliss—which should, however, not be confused with fun. The great myth researcher Joseph Campbell said in this regard: "Follow your bliss. If you do follow your bliss, you put yourself on a kind of track that has been there all the while waiting for you, and the life you ought to be living is the one you are living. Wherever you are—if you are following your bliss, you are enjoying that refreshment, that life within you, all the time". One of my teachers, Oskar Schlag, once told me at a crossroads in my life: "Where there is no joy, there is no path".

> **Shadow diary**
>
> What do I show of myself? How do I behave towards my family, my partner, my friends, colleagues, bosses? What do others expect from me? How do things stand with joy on my path?
>
> Please record your findings and thoughts in your shadow diary.

Danger and Rescue from the Shadow Domain

Fairy tales and myths as signposts

A **danger** that is well recognized by the conservative world is that of getting lost in the shadow realm or surrendering all power to the shadow. When the dark side gains the upper hand—especially after having been mercilessly repressed for a long time—we speak of "psychosis", when it keeps hold of it, of "schizophrenia". Unfortunately, orthodox medicine, casting its magic spell of great fearfulness and resistance with regard to this scenario, ends up amplifying this danger even further. Those who suppress all manifestations of shadow in an uncompromisingly allopathic fashion simply make its sudden eruption into everyday life more likely. A quote from the apocryphal *Gospel of Thomas* (verse 70) points out this connection: "If you bring forth what is within you, what you bring forth will save you. If you do not bring forth what is within you, it will destroy you."

What gets completely overlooked, on the other hand, is the danger of us completely mistaking our persona for our true self. Many people in the modern world consider their mask or façade to be their true self. Nevertheless, when we describe a person as nothing but a mask and therefore hollow and empty, this speaks volumes and reveals how little we think of that person.

The tendency for us to confuse our true self with our outer façade is gaining popularity today. This has become particularly clear in a concrete way with the proliferation of plastic surgery in the service of cosmetic goals. In this respect, everything boils down to appearance, in other words, to nothing more than the facade. As a general rule, the overall functioning of the reworked body regions is usually diminished; the related sense of feeling is ignored entirely. Enlarged breasts, extended limbs, retightened faces or newly-styled vaginas are impaired in their functioning by these surgical operations, which pay no regard to the sensations associated with them. Once again, this is a further example of our typical, modern-day rebellion against our given reality, or in other words, against what is.

At the same time, the mistake of confusing our status with our true self is also running rampant, and many money managers and stock-market fans apparently consider themselves to be their bank account. Such people appear almost *too good to be true*; they are good in a way that seems almost surreal, and in fact they are indeed not real. Those who identify themselves only with parts of their persona, such as their appearance, their clothing, their status in the form of titles or economic power, in the end wind up with something hollow and fake in this respect. In contrast, every part of our shadow that we accept and that as a result is added to our reality makes us more real and all-encompassing. Of course, at the same time, this makes us more ambivalent and multidimensional and thus more profound and more human. The more shadow aspects move from the unconscious to the ego, the more expansive and more open the latter becomes. Consequently, we are also more able to perceive ourselves, our Self and our world as they really are—rather than simply as a projection from our unconscious shadow reality.

But just how is this rescue from the shadow domain, this integration of shadow able to take place? Fairy tales and myths provide the most beautiful and timeless answers here. Many fairy tales, from *The Frog Prince* through to *Beauty and the Beast*, present us with excellent examples of how darkest shadows can be transformed into brightest light. Princes and princesses are cursed in fairy tales by unknown dark creatures and transformed into abysmally-ugly figures. Usually, they must then remain trapped in their repulsive bodies until love redeems them. In effect, this means that someone must recognize their true noble and lovable essence behind the ugly façade and love them despite the ugliness of their physical appearance. In this respect, fairy tales of this sort present us with a reversal of our modern-day situation, in which, behind noble façades, the darkest and ugliest shadows are to be found. Fairy tale characters are mostly forced by their respective curses to openly display their shadow to everyone. The figures in our modern-day fairy tale of progress often live out the darkest shadow behind beautiful artificial façades. Possibly this is the more terrible curse.

Oscar Wilde portrayed this classic theme in his famous novel *The Portrait of Dorian Gray*. The novel tells the story of a beautiful young man whose shadow is removed in a magical game. This is then instead projected onto a painting instead. The portrait now ages on his behalf and even takes on all of his unsightly character traits. The fact that his body remains youthfully beautiful and desirable forever is certainly also the dream of many people in our modern world, who place their salvation in the skilled hands of the surgeons of the beautification industry. In the novel, however, this becomes a nightmare, because at some point, Dorian Gray has to reunite with his shadow. In the end, a repulsively-ugly, old man is found lying dead in front of the painting, which now shows the beautiful young man again.

When it comes to fairy tales, we can assume that all of the characters represent parts of our own soul. In other words, in the case of the beast and the frog prince, the shadow that was long banished to the inner world has gained the upper hand and now becomes visible on the outside. In this respect, this dark, unattractive aspect that has been brought to light is awaiting salvation. For this to occur, it must be accepted and loved by the ego, the conscious part of our own being. When that happens, our shadow reveals a wonderful gift. And it is no accident that for "gift", we also use the word "present", and that the word "present" in turn refers both to the present moment, as well as being present in the moment. In fact, it is in that moment of acceptance in the timeless present that the gift is revealed.

In the fairy tale of *The Frog Prince*, what this means is that the beautiful princess has split off her dark shadow and banished it. It sits as a wet and cold frog in the dark pond, in other words, in the watery realm of the soul. It is into this murky water of all places that her golden ball—the symbol of her Self—falls, which leaves her heartbroken. Now the only way to get back to her golden wholeness leads via the ugly frog. Only he can help her to reach her Self in the form of the golden ball. The frog is also willing to do so; but it demands her love. Nevertheless, the princess does not want to let herself be blackmailed by the frog—and slams it against the wall. At this moment, she stands up for herself, no longer allowing herself to be influenced by the rules and admonitions of her father, and with her authentic stance, ends up releasing the frog, thus making love possible. Her liberated and honest archetypal male aggression releases her shadow, the male part of her soul or her Animus.

Following her confrontation with the shadow, it is love that illuminates the dark shadow and sets it free. In the transcendental "higher psychology"[22] of fairytales, redemption corresponds to the mystical marriage and enlightenment. This is also the case in the fairy tale *Beauty and the Beast,* in which Belle voluntarily returns to the Beast. In other words, the soul returns to the dark aspect that it had split off from itself and reunites with it. The heroine also has to redeem her dark, ugly male aspect.

As in *The Frog Prince*, the wedding is symbolic of the gift that lies in the process of shadow redemption. It is only through the union with the dark side that the relationship and life itself can

---

22 This concept stems from Oskar Ruf in: *Die esoterische Bedeutung der Märchen (The Esoteric Meaning of Fairy tales).* Knaur, München 1996

succeed. This is still the case today and will continue to remain so.

Fairy tales make it clear that love is the only force that can integrate shadow. If all of the characters in a fairy tale can be found in us, the story is actually about love of our Self or self-love. This includes having the courage to stand up for ourselves and to become authentic. This love makes us beautiful and allows us to love others. This is because, from a Christian point of view, we are ideally able to love our neighbor as we love ourselves. Erich Fromm says in his book *The Art of Loving* that love is a creative act of the soul.[23] As a result, when we creatively draw love from our innermost source, then we no longer make a difference between you and me.

The essence of love is a supporting force from within and enables us to open up to others and to accept ourselves. Those who deal successfully with their shadow will be beautiful and light forever. Both the princess and Belle must first accept their own shadow in order to find the most desirable and beautiful thing in this deepest darkness: the love of their life. Therein lies the secret of the gift in the shadow, which will continue to be the focus of our attention.

William Miller writes in his book *Your Golden Shadow*: "We must come face to face with the possible worst in us in order to discover the prospects for a deeper and richer life and a greater fulfillment of self. If we continue to identify and own only the bright side of ourselves (persona), life will be progressively artificial, boring and uncreative."[24] For seekers, there is simply no alternative to the path that is being advocated here in such a compelling way. However, it is by no means without danger. We must be aware of the shadow at every moment and always take it seriously. We should never underestimate it and approach it too rashly or simply blindly let it run free without recognizing it.

---

23 Erich Fromm, *The Art of Loving*. New York: Harper & Row, 1989, ©1956.

24 William A. Miller, *Your Golden Shadow: Discovering and Fulfilling Your Undeveloped Self*. Harper & Row, 1989, pg 69

Being able to look into our own abyss without plunging headlong into it is an important part of what makes us human and underlies our much-cited reputation as Creation's crowning glory.

Whenever seekers have encountered wholeness or unity, they had to protect themselves or ended up suffering great harm. Moses can only perceive Yahweh via the projection of the burning bush. In Greek mythology, a drama always develops when mortals insist on confronting the deity face to face. Miller writes from a psychological point of view: "We could never take the disclosure all at once; it would be absolutely overwhelming—we would be hopelessly destroyed. Sometimes people foolishly proclaim that they want to be absolutely, nakedly honest with themselves—know themselves inside out, nothing held back. This is nothing less than an invitation to insanity. We should not for one minute discount the power of shadow or downplay the possible ramifications of discovery."[25]

The practical work of reincarnation therapy shows how patients with the ugliest shadow experiences do not become repulsive, but instead lovable—for themselves and their environment—as soon as they honestly accept these experiences and thus learn to love them as well. This is also the reason why we accept each and every patient for therapy. As soon as a patient confronts their shadow and becomes honest, they become immensely lovable. The psychoanalytical method of conscious patient selection reveals how comparatively exclusive and therefore shadow-protecting this method is.

In the uncompromising confrontation with our shadow, fairy tales exude a special power. "Children are told fairy tales so that they fall asleep, adults so that they wake up," says the Argentinian psychiatrist and therapist Jorge Bucay. Fairy tales are actually much more than edifying stories for children to read aloud while falling asleep, although they have also proven themselves to be wonderfully effective for this purpose for centuries. Fairy tales contain archetypal basic patterns and wisdom of the soul

25 Ibid Miller, pg 70

and are signposts for human development. In a variety of ways and according to individual needs, they always revolve around the one truth. The psychologist, astrologer and fairy tale specialist Claus Riemann says: "Fairy tales are not real, but they are true. They allow access to the timeless wisdom of the human soul, to archetypal figures and developmental motifs that have been the same in all times and in all cultures and will always be the same."[26]

With this in mind, it is by no means surprising that, in all fairy tales, developmental helpers in the form of shadow figures play an important, and even decisive role. The paths of development in fairy-tales are lined with evil stepmothers, emotionally-cold fathers, witches, the evil wolf or the devil and even his grandmother as well. Without them, development would not get going at all, and no (re)solution would be possible. All of these shadow figures contribute in the sense of Goethe's Mephisto as:

> "part of the power that would
> always wish Evil,
> and always works the Good."

Even though such figures deliberately try to hinder the fairy tale hero, they are in fact the ones who make his progress possible.

What is also astonishing is how strongly the fairy tale heroes are aware of the necessity of shadow figures. They neither blame nor condemn the villains, nor do they moan or complain in the least about the shadow figures. Projection is not an issue for fairy tale heroes. Instead, the significance of the shadow figures for their own destiny is taken seriously.

Only at the end of each fairy tale, i.e. at the end of the path to reach salvation, after the heroes have overcome their "shadow existence" as it were and become completely themselves, do the shadow(figure)s disappear from their lives as if by themselves.

---

26 Claus Riemann, *Alter König—Neuer König: Seelenweisheit im Märchen**. (*Old King—New King: Spiritual wisdom in fairy tales.*) Self-published, 2007.

Until then, the fairy tale heroes face all of the adversities and obstacles that the shadow figures put in their path in a variety of ways. At the same time, exactly the right helpers always join them and stay by their side. These light helper figures also have a connection to the dark (unconscious) areas of the soul, where they embody the inner wealth hidden within the shadow.

Such helpers often take the form of animals. In the fairy tale *Cinderella*, it is the doves that help to distinguish good from bad ("The good ones in the pot, the bad ones in the crop"). Generally speaking, animals bring us into contact with the primal power of our natural instincts. Through the connection to this energy, seemingly unmanageable tasks can easily be solved. For Cinderella, it is all about recognizing what is good (for her). The "bad" is not condemned, but instead taken inward, processed, transformed and excreted or let go of.

The good fairy watching over Cinderella, i.e. the deceased mother as the guardian spirit, shows the extent to which we are guided from beyond. Beyond our normal perception, there is this mysterious other world that takes care of us. The trust that Cinderella places in these inner helpers and the unconditional acceptance of her own "shadow existence" lead her more or less automatically to her true place in life. The shoe that fits her and only her is symbolic of this and sends Cinderella on her way.

In the fairy tale of *Snow White*, envy and jealousy, two dark feelings that often appear in the company of beauty, are the shadows of the evil stepmother. They are a threat to Snow White's life and her intact world. For this reason, the graceful young girl has to flee into the dark, dangerous forest (of the soul) and hide behind the mountains with the seven dwarves. Dwarves also symbolize soul powers that have been banished into the dark. At the same time, they are employees of Pluto-Hades, the ancient god of the Underworld. In his realm, in the dark mines, the dwarves bring his riches to light: the precious gems and metals are symbolic of our own treasures that are buried in the shadow realm. In this case, the dwarves are light helpers who protect Snow White during her stay in the shadow kingdom. Despite all their warnings, however, Snow White must go her own way. The fact that she falls for the evil tricks of the step-motherly witch, (symbol of the dark feminine), three times and still survives, reveals how she never loses her faith and trust in her necessary path. As a result, Snow White is able to be found by the prince (who is always the symbol for the Animus, our inner male component) and to unite with him. And only then does Snow White become whole. From now on, the beauty of her inner Self radiates through her external beauty as well. Consequently, the evil stepmother—the dark female shadow—dies. Snow White has accepted this aspect, suffered through it, and thus shone light upon it, thereby robbing it of the need for its existence. And this step, which unites the light and the dark feminine aspects, prepares the heroine for the next union with her male light shadow, the Animus or king's son.

The tale of *Sleeping Beauty* also follows this same shadow pattern. The thirteenth fairy, who represents death, has not been invited to the feast celebrating the birth of Sleeping Beauty, based on (masculine) rationalist reasoning (i.e. there is not enough tableware). However, she refuses to let herself be excluded. The longing for immortality, or the fear of death, are primal human instincts. Nevertheless, death is an unavoidable part of our life on this earthly plane. A mother gives birth to a child, but also gives its future death to it at the same time. Thirteen is considered an unlucky number because it is symbolically connected with these dark aspects of the feminine. Friday the 13th has such a bad reputation because it additionally refers to the day of the week which was dedicated to the Germanic goddess Freyja. The attempt to escape from this darkest part of our life is the subject of many stories, for example, in *Godfather Death* when the godson plays games with the Grim Reaper trying to bargain for a longer lifetime. But, in this case as well, it is important to face this aspect and to integrate it into our life.

The exclusion of the thirteenth fairy in the fairy tale of Sleeping Beauty leads, as it were, to a life that is akin to a stunned state of deep sleep. In the end, the fairy's curse inevitably takes effect. Despite all of the precautions taken by the king, who has sought his salvation in the functional measure of burning all the spindles in the land, Sleeping Beauty still ends up pricking herself on a spindle, and then falls into a deathlike slumber. Together with Sleeping Beauty, the whole kingdom descends into a deep sleep, too. The castle becomes overgrown with thorny hedges, i.e. vitality is lacking; the flow of life has been halted. The fear of death paralyses everyone. It was supposed to have been banished, but it is precisely because of this, that everyone has fallen into this state of suspended animation. The bottom line is this: we can only really achieve true vitality and quality of life if we become aware of the shadow of death, i.e. the finiteness of our life, and fully accept it as a part of our existence.

What would life look like if it never ended? An endless series of days filled with trivialities would stretch before us. The finiteness of our life is thus a wise gift. It forces us to savour every moment. And it is a gracious gift, because we can start over and over again. This thought is also echoed in the fairy tale. After a hundred years of deep slumber, Sleeping Beauty may awaken again, but only after her (inner) prince has acknowledged and conquered the polarity of life. The young man has the courage to penetrate the dense, thorn-spiked hedge and to free Sleeping Beauty from her "ideal-world magic spell". The pain, the thorns, belong to life, as does death.

In the fairy tale *Little Red Riding Hood*, we find the well-meaning mother who wants to protect her child by warning her not to leave the (right and thus archetypically-male) path. In modern terms, this means that Little Red Riding Hood is supposed to adapt to the current social norms and follow the mainstream. This path may seem safe, but it prevents Little Red Riding Hood's individual development.

In the form of the evil wolf, Little Red Riding Hood finds a (seductive) leader, who takes her on the path to individuation. As is so often the case, we encounter shadow in the form of the wolf in sheep's clothing. Suspecting nothing and with childlike naivety, Little Red Riding Hood instinctively lays the groundwork for the wolf, who subsequently familiarizes her with life in the world of opposites in the form of the polarity of good and evil. It is on her way through the dark forest of her soul that the girl gets to know life in the first place and finds (soul)mates. She thereby frees herself from the narrowly-limited realm of her norm-abiding family. When she finally reaches her grandmother's house, it is not a protective grandmother who awaits her. Instead, she finds the wolf, who is pretending to be her grandmother, and who is thus trying to act as meek as a lamb.

Little Red Riding Hood is frightened by the dangerous and threatening appearance of her grandmother's shadow. Nevertheless, in her as yet still carefree child-like state, she allows herself to be fully drawn into the events—and is devoured by the evil wolf. Symbolically, she embarks on a journey into the shadow realm. It is only in the belly of the wolf that she again meets the protective female soul component that is represented by the grandmother.

Help and salvation are also provided here by a male (Animus) figure: the hunter. He also acts as an ally of the shadow kingdom. He has a close relationship with the instinctive forces of nature, in particular with the animals, which he kills on the one hand, but nourishes and cherishes on the other. In this respect, he unites these two contrasting aspects of living in a world of polarity in a non-judgemental and neutral way. Instead of just the food for children (i.e. cake), which we find in Little Red Riding Hood's basket of provisions, as a hunter, he also brings "carnal food" into the game of life. With a courageous cut, he frees Little Red Riding Hood and her grandmother from the wolf's womb. Through this aggressive act (of birth) in the sense of a fairy-tale Caesarean section, the previously protected little girl symbolically becomes a woman who now knows both sides of life. The dark shadow is, of course, represented in the animalistic devouring by the wolf, the light shadow in the hunter who frees her.

In the fairy tale *Rumpelstiltskin*, we meet the shadow in the form of the boastful father, who brags that his daughter can spin straw into gold. The king, who is greedy for gold, then has the girl locked up in a chamber, where she is to prove the existence of this gift overnight. In this way, the shadow, here in the form of masculine greed for recognition and ever more possessions, sets the process of development in motion.

In this fairy tale, there is also a figure from the shadow realm who appears as a helper: Rumpelstiltskin. Embodying a mixture of nature spirit and the devil's co-worker, he twice spins the straw into gold for our fairy-tale heroine, after she promises him her dearest possessions as a reward. Each of these is a memento from the past that she is attached to. Symbolically, she is thereby called upon to sacrifice and let go of the old, or in other words, to let go of the past.

> ## Shadow diary
>
> What is or was my favourite fairy tale? Read it again, or better still: have someone read it to you.
>
> What does it say about my shadow, or in other words, how is the role of evil expressed in it? If this time round, I experience all of the characters of the fairy tale once again as parts of my soul, what does my fairy tale tell me?
>
> Please record your thoughts and insights in your shadow diary.

Nevertheless, the king's greed only increases with all the gold, and when the young woman has nothing left to give, she has to promise Rumpelstiltskin her dearest asset in the future—her first child—in order to save her life. Consequently, she makes a pact and pledges away her future, thereby suppressing the threatening consequences of her actions (into the shadows).

Enthusiastic about her extraordinary abilities, the king takes her as his wife and soon after their first child is born. Now the time has come to honor the pact with the shadow devil. And as is so often the case in normal, less fairy tale-like life, this is when the negotiations begin. Pleading and begging, she tries to pull her head out of the agreement noose. And once again, Rumpelstiltskin is prepared to make a deal; as a shadow (figure), he wants more than anything to be acknowledged and recognized. This is symbolically expressed in the fact that the fairy-tale heroine has to find out his real name in order for Rumpelstiltskin to set her free.

Calling something by its name always entails acknowledging it. As a result, a grand collection of all possible names is carried out throughout the kingdom. But, of course, the right shadow name cannot be found in the familiar, external world. Instead, it is overheard from Rumpelstiltskin himself in the darkness of the night, and thus the spell is broken.

Rumpelstiltskin disintegrates as a shadow because he has been acknowledged and recognized. In the fairy tale as a whole, however, this particular shadow figure was actually the great helper who set the heroine on her way. Corresponding shadow transformations can be found in countless fairy tales across the most diverse cultures throughout the world. Time and time again, we come across the same pattern. The shadow is "necessary" in the original sense of this word. Stemming from *ne-* "not" + *cedere* "to withdraw", it meant "no backing away". It is by confronting the shadow rather than "backing away" from it that we can find our very own and at the same time primeval human path of development. The shadow is our source of strength, our ally and represents the task that we have to undertake. Like one of the enchanted fairy-tale creatures, it longs for recognition, illumination and redemption.

Shadow qualities

Since all unlived aspects of life become shadow, shadow topics are by no means only dark and negative. Jeremiah Abrams, an American shadow therapist, sees this as his task, "... to give reality and meaning to what may be working through a client, to help them become more aware of the denied parts of themselves. The greatest sin may be the unlived life."[27]

"The fact that I didn't really live my own life"—this is the "sin" that people on their deathbeds actually regret far more than any mistakes they might have made. There are three things that they wish for most of all: to have lived more, to have taken more risks, and to have exercised more discipline. What stopped them was fear. Fear is one of the greatest sources of shadow; anxiety therapies are therefore an effective form of shadow treatment.[28]

When all is said and done, all of the shortcomings that they are expressing such regret about amount to having devoted too little attention to the Self and thus to the integration of the shadow. A result of this is that, in conventional society, even such wonderful aspects as ecstasy and orgiastic sexuality easily slip into the shadows, where they wait for liberation. In a similar vein, emotionality, sensitivity and love sink readily into the shadow realm. Our own strength and competence, authenticity and genuineness, our genius and the undiscovered artist in ourselves also often get buried early in life, because they lead to us rubbing others the wrong way. Shadow is simply everything that we would never do, but would have loved to do and should now definitely do after all. Anyone who has countless heroes and idols—regardless of which domain they perform in—is projecting positive qualities onto these stars in the external world.

Ultimately, we must become like our idols and ensure that we are able to realize within ourselves the illuminating and fascinating star qualities that allow our idols to stand out in an outstanding way. Those who become heroes in their own lives in this way need fewer heroes in the external world, and such heroes then take on a lower status for them. As soon as you realize your own dreams and visions, you no longer have to project them onto other dreamers and visionaries. If you are a football

---

27 In the preface to Debbie Ford: *The Dark Side of the Light Chasers*, loc. cit., p. xiv

28 For example with the help of the program Angstfrei Leben (Living an anxiety-free life*) (Book and CD)

Shadow diary

Do I have idols? Are there heroes in the sports world or show business stars that I admire? Who do I adore, who do I worship like a god? How many and what sort of wishes do I still have?

Please note your answers in your shadow diary.

star yourself, you are unlikely to travel to see other football stars as a fan. Pop stars usually don't go round acting as the groupies of other pop idols.

Great wisdom lies in the saying of the Hasidic rabbi Susya shortly before his death: "When I go to heaven, they won't ask me: 'Why weren't you Moses? But they will ask, 'Why weren't you Susya? Why didn't you become what only you could become?'"

Far less suspicious than idols when it comes to shadow are role models. This is because they can promote development in a positive way. Those who emulate a great role model will neither copy that person's life, nor constantly want to follow them on their travels, nor, for example, try to gain insights about that person and participate in their life by reading the gossip pages. Instead, they will live their own life and follow that person's example. They want to realize qualities of the role model in themselves and must develop accordingly. On the other hand, anyone who virtually avoids their own life in order to align it entirely with their idol is simply projecting positive qualities onto another. They do everything in their power to constantly sit at the feet of their idol, and do little to develop the idolized traits within themselves. Nevertheless, this latter process is necessary in order to take back the projection and grow up.

Just as we need a list of our negative shadow aspects in order to grow towards our full potential, a list of our positive shadow aspects is also essential. All of our dreams, desires and visions long for realization and contain positive shadow aspects that are yearning to be brought to life and recognized. Anyone or anything we have admired in our lives up till now—can be of help in putting together a list of positive shadow aspects of this type.

Practical Exercise

Start keeping a list in your shadow diary of positive and negative qualities. Everything that you admire goes on the first list, everything that you reject and condemn gets put on the second one.

List the concepts or key words on the left side of the page so that there is enough room on the right for further notes. Later you can add in the opposite pole here, which will provide you with further realizations.

For the practical exercise of fulfilling our own dreams and wishes, we certainly do not need to wait until our time is almost up, as is the case in the *wonder*-ful film *The Bucket List*. In this film, Jack Nicholson and Morgan Freeman play two older, seriously-ill cancer patients, who shortly before they are about to "kick the bucket" set about writing down all of their remaining dreams on a list and making these come true. In the rest of the film, they work through this so-called "bucket list" in a very charming way. In the process, they soon realize how much quality life still holds for them, even though their good health has long since vanished. In line with the motto "There is a life before death", it would, of course, be of even more benefit to create a list of this type much earlier in life.

It is also worth keeping in mind that, at the end of a so-called "good" and even particularly "respectable" life, it is more than possible that a model citizen may knock on the pearly gates and still be refused entry, because he missed out on 783 mind-blowing orgasms and over 1,000 average ones, 445 moments of intoxicated rapture and 789 experiences of great ecstasy, hundreds of orgies celebrated with wild abandon and 4,598 moments of idle bliss with no deeper meaning, 34,876 loving looks into children's eyes filled with wonder and 8,456 touching moments of deep empathy with animals and even deeper ones with other people. And it could be much worse or even so much more pleasant, but it is, of course, difficult to imagine that the guardian of this threshold is such a pedantic bean counter.

There is very little in life that we have practised so thoroughly as the processes of assessing and judging value, and then in the end passing judgement and being judgemental. We can therefore make good use of our expertise in this respect in order to use well-known and well-worn paths to get closer to our shadow. So, by all means, feel free to once again make value judgements and be judgemental to your heart's content as a good way to finding your own shadow.

As far as dealing with negative judgements are concerned, a great sense of relief results from having learned to first recognize our positive sides and praise ourselves for them beforehand. Those who have learned to accept themselves in a positive way and to be proud of their own achievements are naturally able to accept their shadow aspects more easily. The lives of such people display greater equilibrium and they are not constantly in danger of being thrown off balance. The best way to get started with recognizing our own achievements is by filling out a balance sheet for our own life.

Film Meditation

Watch the film *The Bucket List*, and as the film credits start to roll to the tune of John Mayer's "Say", allow your eyes in the outer world to close. As you ease deeper and deeper into a state of relaxation, let all of the accomplishments and successes in your life that have led you to this point of uniqueness emerge before your inner eye.

Ask yourself: What do I find wonderful about myself—and others? How and from what point onwards do I want to realize these qualities in myself?

And right now, create your own list in the form of inner images of all those things you still want to achieve, realize and experience in this life, including all those destinations you still want to visit, the dreams that still live within your soul, the desires and longings that you still feel.

Afterwards, transfer everything to your shadow diary, where your list will then take shape. And start working through this list as quickly as you can, straightaway or the coming weekend at the latest, or in any case, during your next vacation.

Transforming challenges into gifts

If we –just for the sake of practice—start actively judging our fellow humans and our environment to our heart's content, we will find it easy to draw up a list of all the terrible things that we dislike in the outside world. What bothers us the most (about ourselves and others) is then given a high ranking and minor vices and problems are put at the bottom of the list. By working like the devil to put items on our negative list, we end up listing things that necessarily have to do with us.

All our handicaps, negative aspects and ugly sides are by their very nature actually challenges. When they were initially not accepted by our environment in the shop display window of our lives and we couldn't find any takers for them, we removed them from the shelves and put them under the counter. We then, of course, remained stuck with them. And at some point in our lives, we will suddenly happen upon this collection, this stockpile of unpopular items. We can, however, choose to deal with it now in a conscious way and of our own free will. This also allows us to be enriched by everything in the outside world that we currently dislike simply because it seems so foreign to our nature, but that actually belongs to us, too. As has already been mentioned, it is here that we guard our greatest and most valuable treasures. They lie buried in a place where, up until now, we probably would have least expected to find them, namely very close to us and centrally located, in the heart of our very being and in the dark.

The list of negative characteristics should be really substantial and complete. And it will end up that way as long as we don't falsely impose any constraints upon ourselves. Once the list is completed, we can examine these characteristics for their redeeming qualities against the background of polarity and can thereby direct the light of consciousness onto them. By cultivating this game of transformation in this way, shadows become treasures. The more redeemed shadow side of perfectionism and obsessiveness, for example, is integrity and flawlessness. In the same way, narrow-minded miserliness gives rise to the potential gain of taking meaningful and useful precautions in keeping with the old saying: "Waste not, want not". On the whole, it is not a case of trying to eradicate dark sides and force them out of our lives forever, but rather of drawing them back in and thereby recognizing and integrating the positive aspects they encompass. The longer and more daunting our negative list is, the greater and more beautiful the gifts that can be derived from it.

In doing so, there are a manageable number of principles that we now want to go into in more detail. We can access these with the help of inner images, but also via intellectual understanding. Those who are aware of these principles and know how to apply them in practice generally have it much easier in life. The great opportunity that this brings with it goes far beyond just finding the treasure in each shadow problem. Knowledge of these principles enables resolutions to be successfully put into practice, projects to be realised and real prevention to be undertaken.

A simple example can help to make this clear: fits of rage and angry outbursts are a shadow topic. At a deeper level, however, it is possible to recognize underlying forms of energy that are extremely helpful. Those who are familiar with the archetypal world can immediately look to what is behind the (original) principle of aggression. Its more redeeming variants include courage, decisiveness, high energy and strength. These can be released from anger and rage and put to good use for a more complete life. This is the idea behind a book like *Aggression as an Opportunity** (see reference list).

This is not the only topic for which it is possible to see many more aspects for both sides of the principle. Brutality is obviously not a redeeming characteristic, but assertiveness is its corresponding redeemed side. Both sides lie opposite each other and complement each other at the same time. The darker the shadow aspect on the one side, the brighter the gift on the other side. This game can be carried on in the same way for all of the principles that constitute reality. Ugliness belongs to the shadow domain—its basis is disharmony. On the opposite side lies beauty. This polarity becomes clear in the fairytale *Beauty and the Beast*. This means that, in all forms of disharmony, there is also the opportunity for harmony.

Just how profound this game with the principles truly is can already be clearly seen at this point. Not only does each archetype have redeemed and unredeemed sides in and of itself, but the various archetypes also lie opposite each other forming natural counterpoles. Clearly, war and the principle of aggression represent the natural opposite to peace. We see this in ancient Roman and Greek mythology when Venus (Aphrodite) and Mars (Ares) join forces and bear children like Concordia (Harmonia) and Cupid (Eros). True harmony and true eroticism need both sides of reality in the form of dynamic masculine energy and gentle feminine energy. Nevertheless, the two gods also bear two shadow children—the twin brothers Timor (Phobos) and Formido (Deimos). Of course, these in turn also conceal light sides in their shadow: in the case of Phobos and the fears he represents, it is expansiveness that forms the natural opposite to narrowness and constriction. The positive sides of Deimos' demonic world were already covered in the beginning chapters. In a similar vein, the American Buddhist and psychiatrist, Edward Podvoll, initially called his wonderful book on the shadow realm in psychiatry, (which was quoted previously) *The Seduction of Madness*. At a later point, publishers who were more hostile to the concept of shadow preferred to give it the title *Recovering Sanity*. Seen from the polar perspective on life, however, the first title does more justice to the book.

A further topic that casts many different shadows is that of "reduction to the essential", which in mythological terms is linked to Saturn. Illness belongs to this topic, too, because it cuts us down to size and limits us, catapulting us back to what is essential. In the sense of *The Healing Power of Illness*, this can become a gift if we are able to discover its other redeemed side.

For its role in propelling us back to the fundamental questions of human existence, illness should actually always be seen as a gift. Starting from a common basis of reduction to the essential, the myriad different symptoms associated with the innumerable different possible clinical pictures can be classified as subcategories of broader themes. In more complex clinical pictures, a combination of different themes can be identified. This is what underlies the method of interpreting the deeper meaning of specific illnesses, as presented in the reference work *Disease as a Symbol* (see footnotes).

The principle of "reduction to the essential" also applies to the aspect of "work", which for many seems to be a negative shadow aspect, but for others provides a great deal of pleasure and meaning to their lives instead. The harshness of life may be counted as shadow, but well-defined structures as light; strictness and severity as shadow, but consistency as light.

Similarly, when it comes to the principle of "exchange and communication", both empty gossip and vital information lie at opposite ends of the same polarity. Pompous grandeur, on the one hand, and benevolent largesse and tolerance, on the other, are both to be found in the archetype of "expansion and growth". Boastful bragging and the natural radiance of a winning personality show two different sides of the same central archetypal principle of the Sun. Snappishness and clamming shut when insulted or showing deep empathy and devotion towards others are two sides of the same archetypal Moon principle that includes both motherliness and childhood innocence, and rhythm as well.

We should therefore never forget that each and every negative side has its positive counterpart. An electric shock can kill—and save lives—when used, for example, in the medical treatment of heart murmurs, as is the case with defibrillation. Snake venom can just as easily cost lives as save them. A deity like the Indian goddess Kali brings forth life and later devours it again in the end. Following in her wake, every mother gives life to a child at birth but also gives birth to that child's eventual death at the same time. In her books, *Goddesses in Everywoman* and *Gods in Everyman*[29], the author Jean Shinoda Bolen has touched upon the whole spectrum of the gods with their two

29 Jean Shinoda Bolen, Harper Collins 1984, 20th anniversary edition, 2004, 30th anniversary edition, 2014); *Gods in Everyman: Archetypes that Shape Men's Lives* (HarperCollins 1989, 25th anniversary edition, 2014)

sides. These are implanted in seed form in each and every one of us and simply lie dormant waiting to be allowed to grow. The shadow is the dark topsoil for these gods, topics or principles. It is up to us to let them into our consciousness and to enrich our lives with their energy. And our soul knows a wonderful way to gain access to them—via inner images.

Meditation

Read Meditations 1 & 9 aloud to yourself.

You can repeat this meditation as often as you like until all of the topics that seem important to you have been transformed.

Twelve archetypal rooms of Light and Shadow

Returning to the image, which has already been used several times, of life as a kind of shop, with a window display, in which we offer the different parts of ourselves as products, it was previously noted that experiences in the first half of life lead to an increasingly limited range being on offer and to a growing number of unpopular, hard-to-sell items forming a shadow collection. Another way to think about this offering is to classify it in terms of twelve inner rooms. These, for example, are like twelve spacious double rooms in a giant mansion that we move into at the same time and in the same way that we move into the temple of our body when we are conceived. At the beginning of life, each of the double rooms lies in bright sunlight, and we have unlimited access to all of the rooms.

Over time, however, wild vines start to creep up along the walls, increasingly overgrowing the windows, with the result that there is less and less light and more and more shadow in the rooms. We live in this house from the very beginning, playing, learning and growing in it. Over time, we learn that those areas that sink into the darkness of the unconscious are dirty and impure and are therefore to be avoided. Everything that frightens us and that we push into the unconscious for this reason also ends up getting dumped on top of this. Gradually, large sections and sometimes even whole rooms sink into oblivion in this way, buried under a layer of dust and cobwebs. All of these still exist of course; they simply no longer play a role in our normal daily consciousness and everyday life. By the time they reach adolescence, some people find themselves living in just one or two remaining rooms; the rest of them have largely been put into mothballs. The people concerned simply no longer enter many of these rooms, and at some point, they will even forget that they even exist. And often, they may then even forget that they have forgotten them, and when that happens, their world becomes small and narrow once and for all.

If we forget who we are and who we could be, that is bad enough. But if we also forget that we have forgotten it, we become separated not only from our original potential, but from all future possibilities as well.

In effect, we start with a large, open mansion, which over time deteriorates into a kind of closed-up shadow palace if, more often than not, vitality is simply allowed to slip through the cracks from many of the rooms. Many people may have been more obedient to their parents, teachers, and their environment, while others were less so and more curious as a result. But each of us has the chance to reclaim our mansion and to not only turn its shadow-filled ruins back into a wonderful and grand house, but also into a palace in a very positive sense as the temple of the evolved soul. If we direct our consciousness into all twelve rooms, which each represent an important principle, and we make the best of each room with the help of this awareness, we can finally live in the castle of our consciousness, and in the fullness of our possibilities.

The following division of the qualities and characteristics of each of these principles into strengths and weaknesses is not to be understood as a value judgement in the usual sense. Since we assume that everything that is unconscious belongs to the shadow, both weaknesses and strengths can be unconscious and thus can end up locked away in the shadow domain.

1. *New beginnings, aggression*

Strength/task: energy and drive, decisiveness, activity, initiative, willpower, development of character, assertiveness, spontaneity, moral courage, breaking new ground, forging new pathways and exploring them.

Weakness/shadow: Anger, rage, violence, brutality, competitiveness, lack of self-control, aggressiveness, rashness, elbow mentality, mindless militancy, destruction, territorial disputes, inconsideration, egoism.

2. *Self-esteem, deep-rootedness, sensual pleasure*

Strength/task: establishing inner and outer values, sense of community, upholding what is good, safeguarding the tried and tested, sensual pleasure, loyalty, security, pragmatism, realism, patience, down-to-earth groundedness, closeness to nature, serenity, safety.

Weakness/shadow: Greed, overindulgence, obsession with wealth and possessions, exaggerated striving for material security, imbalance between giving and taking, inertia, stubbornness, sluggishness.

3. *Communication, exchange*

Strength/task: imparting information, gift for languages, neutrality, flexibility, intellect, versatility, logical thinking, sociability, ability to learn, openness, receptiveness, quick grasp of new concepts.

Weakness/shadow: superficiality, opportunism, love of gossip and idle chatter, refined cunning, deceptiveness, lying, swindling, craftiness, sensation-seeking curiosity, fragmentation, doubt, lack of a clear stance, projection, shrewdness, inconsistency.

4. *Sensibility, emotion, sense of security, rhythm of life*

Strength/task: compassion, tender loving care, empathy, helpfulness, nurturance, motherliness, sensitivity, empathy, strong sense of family, spiritual identity, yielding softness. **Weakness/shadow:** melodramatics, sentimentality, emotional neediness, dependency, moodiness, self-pity, emotional blackmail by taking on the victim role, depression, regression, acting like a little child, emotional selfishness, timidity, soppiness, weepiness.

5. *Creativity, charisma, centeredness*

Strength/task: self-expression, authenticity, balance, self-confidence, generosity, joie de vivre, authority, organizational talent, sovereignty, kindness, warm-heartedness, courage, self-reliance, creative intelligence, generosity, genuine warmth and openheartedness.

Weakness/shadow: Egotism, high-handedness, diva-/pasha-like airs and graces, arrogance, boasting, lust for fame, lust for power, lust for prestige, overambition, smugness, craving for adulation, more shadow than substance, conceit ("Me up there, and the underlings below").

6. *Order, reason*

Strength/task: adaptability to existing life circumstances, good powers of observation, economic(al) thinking and behaviour, good discrimination abilities, sensible and efficient planning, accuracy, attention to detail, service, humility, mindfulness, appreciation of small everyday things, work as pleasure.

Weakness/shadow: Criticism, nagging, condemnation, pedantry, splitting hairs, disparagement of others, efficiency at the expense of emotion and vitality, acting only in accordance with overall purpose and potential benefit, losing oneself in unimportant details, distrust, anxiety, hypochondria, stuffiness, being a know-it-all, total obedience to rationality, narrow-mindedness, blind faith in science.

7. *Harmony, partnership, aesthetics*

Strength/task: sense of love, sense of beauty, sense of style, sense of balance, well-roundedness, self-love, finding the way from outer beauty to inner beauty, ability to relate to others, finding joy in contact with others, inner and outer peace, tactfulness, ability to compromise, diplomacy, aesthetics.

Weakness/shadow: false harmony, the beautiful facade, the soulless mask, vanity, falsehood, dishonesty, resentment, expecting others to preserve one's own illusion of a safe and ideal world; addiction to falling in love again and again instead of fully living partnership; fickleness, indecision, half-heartedness, pathological conflict avoidance.

8. *Radical transformation*

Strength/task: ability to adapt and transform, total commitment, willingness to plunge into the deepest depths, regenerative power, daily experience of the death-and-rebirth process, unconditional devotion to a cause, surpassing oneself and outgrowing previous limitations, repentance, change of attitude, conversion and turn-around, confrontation of self and shadow; heading bravely into the unknown to learn the true meaning of "fear"; taking leave again and again, letting go; deep passion.

Weakness/shadow: Destructiveness, obsession, revenge, self-hatred, manipulation, abuse of power, power struggles, jealousy, fanaticism, fixation, dogmatic adherence to principles, relentlessness, back-stabbing, cynicism, sadism, masochism, black-and-white "Either-Or" attitude, total excessiveness or extreme self-denial, emotional vampirism, creating bondage and dependence for others or being enslaved oneself.

9. *Growth, finding meaning in life*

Strength/task: the search for meaning and purpose in life, inner growth, inner abundance and fulfilment, broadening horizons, tolerance, justice (aligning oneself with what is right and true), sense of purpose, ability to synthesize information and maintain the overview, making connections and building bridges between ideas, generosity, in-sight, enthusiasm, finding the right balance, education and wisdom, capacity for faith, religiousness, ethics.

Weakness/shadow: gluttony, never getting enough, immodesty, megalomania, excessiveness, overshooting the mark, wastefulness, addiction to missionizing, condescension, unreasonable and egotistical expansion, self-righteousness, craving for adulation; fear of showing weakness and puniness and being laid bare; excessive exaggeration, hypocrisy, "holier-than-thou" attitude, moral superiority, presumptuous infallibility, arrogant elitism.

10. *Structure, concentration on the essentials*

Strength/task: Narrowing things down to the essence/the essential, clarity, modesty, mastery, ability to concentrate, awareness of tradition, joyful pride in duty, seriousness, reliability, dutifulness, awareness and acceptance of *the Laws of Fate*, conscientiousness, responsibility for oneself, diligence, consistency and perseverance, facing up to consequences, conscious overcoming of obstacles, maturity.

Weakness/shadow: Harshness, strictness, coldness, mercilessness, rigidity, "normopathy" (compulsion to follow rules in order to be considered normal), compulsiveness, blind belief in authority, submissive bowing and scraping, blinker mentality, fear, stinginess, lack of understanding, elevating one's own opinion to the level of the law, grouchiness, lack of feeling, performance as the measure of all things, blocking the flow of life.

11. *Independence, originality*

Strength/task: individualism, liberation from dependencies, union of opposites, objectivity, search for truth, truthfulness, eagerness to experiment, inventiveness, idealism (freedom, equality, brotherliness), developing positive outlooks for the future, finding unconventional solutions, ingenuity, resourcefulness, quick wit, "have-your-cake-and-eat-it-too" attitude towards life, liberality and generosity.

Weakness/shadow: pursuit of life-endangering theories and ideas, cold-blooded struggle for particular ideologies, devaluation of emotion and closeness, eccentricity, rebellion as a matter of principle, constant opposition, pushing through innovation at all costs and without considering the consequences, arrogance, lack of pragmatism, lack of grounding; pretentious belief in one's own specialness; demanding special treatment, becoming an eccentric, anarchy, detachment, exaggerated opinion of oneself.

12. *Dissolution of boundaries*

Strength/task: sense of basic trust, capacity for devotional surrender, sensitivity, mediality, spirituality, intuition, altruism, powers of premonition, ability to sense the reality behind the visible world, boundlessness, cosmic universal love, being at one with everything, spiritual care, capacity for making sacrifices, creative imagination, visionary "big picture" view, compassion; belief, hope, love.

Weakness/shadow: Instability, chaos, repression, head buried in the sand approach, self-deception, living a lie; fleeing from reality, self-delusion; living in fantasy worlds, secretiveness, smoke screens, surrending to addiction instead of undertaking life's quest, losing one's way to the point of madness, helper syndrome, unrealistic dreams, loss of identity, lack of self-confidence, eternal sacrifice, chameleon-like illusory adaptation, seductibility; domination by others, vagueness and lack of contours; unrealised longings.

Meditation

Read Meditations 1 & 10 aloud to yourself.

From your list of negative qualities (Practical exercise on page 138), bring the point that is currently most important into awareness and hold it in your mind's eye. Then allow yourself to sink into a state of relaxation in the usual way, while remaining conscious of your negative point. In this way, whenever you have time and feel the need, you can work through your list of negatives, point by point, in many subsequent meditations and thus resolve everything on the list. At the end of all of this, you will be left with a polarity list on which each shadow aspect is complemented by the respective light

Gathering gifts

In addition to the intuitive path via image meditation, we can also allow the intellect to "work" on the transformation of shadow aspects into gifts, by once again making use of the list of principles.

1. *New beginnings, aggression:* Deep beneath the surface of unbridled aggression, brutality, violence and recklessness, we find strength and courage, along with calm and collected power, and thus even the courage to be gentle. In this way, rough brutality can produce the gift of gentleness. It is perhaps in courage, i.e. the rage of the heart, the lionheart bravado, that the transformed energy becomes most obvious. Deep beneath the surface of impatience lies the possibility of finding quick solutions in cases of emergency, and at the opposite pole, the chance to learn patient endurance.

2. *Self-esteem, deep-rootedness, sensual pleasure:* without being aware of it, the money-obsessed stock exchange

afficionado constantly refines his intuition in line with the curves of the stock exchange. These curves have long since come to mean the world to many men, and as such, have become more important to them than the curves of the female body. With wise foresight regarding future developments, the afficionado can be of use to himself and his family, and in this way, avoid disappointment and misfortune. On the shadow side of his addiction to profit, the insatiably greedy man is forced via his losses to learn to be content, and in doing so, to become modest.

3. *Communication, exchange:* The gossip and the chatterbox can learn to use their form of addictive communication to exchange information and establish common ground. In this way, an addiction to gossiping includes the gift of communion. Travelling salesmen used to carry around a lot of important information in addition to their material offerings. Informants and pimps establish contacts, which can take on the character of a gift. The former provide information, the latter sex. They could shift their creativity to a higher level at any time. Dishonesty and deceitfulness require ingenuity, cunning and selfishness. These facilitate the gifts of refinement and intelligence.

4. *Sensibility, emotion, sense of security, rhythm of life:* Heavy drinkers who view the world through beer goggles to make it more attractive are usually too soft for the harsh world of reality. The gift behind boozing is the desire for softness and security and the ability to empathize and become one with everything.

5. *Creativity, charisma, centeredness:* Puffed up windbags whose words gush out like an endless stream of foam are unpleasant at first glance. However, a closer look reveals the gift that this foam provides—after all, Venus-Aphrodite—the goddess of love—was also born from foam. As a matter of fact, compliments often need a little bit of foam on top just like a good cappuccino or a freshly tapped beer.

6. *Order, reason:* Badly thrown together "tinkering" and handicrafts include the gift of improvisational talent and sustainable help for oneself and others. Stinginess and extreme thrift

can allow the building up of reserves and provisions for the future. Those who quit and turn tail easily can provide the gift of caution and consideration. In this way, they avoid useless arguments and fights, and consequently also injuries and defeats.

7. *Harmony, partnership, aesthetics:* Obscenely dolled-up whores, whose appearance seems embarrassing, can convey the gift of sensuality and eroticism, thereby symbolizing seduction and scintillation and thus also the turn on. The puritanical guardian of virtue who, soured by an overdose of morality, fights against the porn industry while "devouring" one porn movie after the other as part of the surveillance effort, could instead treat himself to the gift of lust and make himself happy. In the shadow of puritanism, it is, of course, unlived lust that lies dormant.

8. *Radical transformation:* In their auto-aggression, self-destructive personalities may recognize the power of radical self-analysis followed by transformation and a change of direction, and in this respect, the magic that lies in the great gift of metamorphosis.

9. *Growth, finding meaning in life:* Those prone to missionizing or being holier-than-thou will discover in their bigotry their longing for faith and (a reconnection to) religion and can start by bestowing this gift upon themselves.

10. *Structure, concentration on the essentials:* In the depths of their obsession, neat freaks and those displaying other compulsive behaviour can learn to recognize their love of structure and trusted values and to give this gift to themselves and the world.

11. *Independence, originality:* Eccentrics and wacky people should recognize the traces of genius and inspiration in their own craziness and zany ideas and thus enrich themselves and the world with these.

12. *Dissolution of boundaries:* In the depths of grumpiness, it is dis-illusion-ment that is to be found. If this is recognized as the end of the "illusion", satisfaction can take its place and be accepted as a gift. Those who cloud things with smoke screens, the many cover-up experts and the daydreamers all

hide mysticism and visions in the depths of their unfathomable souls that this world is desperately yearning for.

Shining lights and villains, provocative topics

Over time—if you want to make intensive use of the practical exercise on page 138—you will fill the lists of positive and negative qualities in your shadow diary with more and more provocative topics. On top of this, deliberately add well-known personalities from history and contemporary public life. In doing so, you may find it equally difficult to admit that you have both the same wonderful qualities as Mahatma Gandhi and the same gruesome qualities as Adolf Hitler. Nevertheless, we will indeed have all of them within us, and this is most definitely the case if these historical figures move us to strong emotional reactions. The matching qualities will certainly be there, but not to the same extent and not on the same level.

In addition, it is, of course, frightening to discover something about ourselves that we have pushed as far away as possible up to this point. At the same time, given the impetus for growth and the treasures contained within it, this provocative topic could actually become a source of joy from now on. The following story may illustrate this point: An artist friend of mine lived in an apartment in an old building equipped with designer furniture and highly-exclusive art, in which a cool and elegant atmosphere prevailed. It was no coincidence that there didn't seem to be a single cosy corner in the whole apartment. A stylish, but uncomfortable sofa, which had obviously been chosen for purely aesthetic, and certainly not for practical reasons, stood in its accustomed place. One day, however, his girlfriend divulged the great secret that the apartment was hiding. Every Saturday evening, when those in the world of his conservative enemies would set off to engage in all sorts of intolerably stuffy, conservative middle-class activities, my artist friend would allow himself to let his hair down and open up a quasi secret chamber in which there was a saggy old sofa. Here he would flop himself down in front of the television to watch the national league football matches on the sports channelwhile drinking beer from cans—and woe betide anyone should disturb him. How much easier it would have been for him to simply allow this part of himself to participate openly in his life. Later, once he'd become an established artist with much greater recognition, he became more relaxed. His mockery of his fellow conservative, middle-class friends diminished, and his soul expanded and allowed cosiness to take its place. He experienced that "cosy" didn't have to have anything to do with "stuffy", even if "stuffy" is often "cosy". Stuffiness can therefore provide the gift of cosiness.

Now is also a good time to consciously consider which general topics and groups of people or professions trigger aggression or rejection in you: Why do Mafia bosses upset you so much? What bothers you about authorities and hierarchies? What about bonuses for bankers? Why do you want to pillory this particular politician or that one? What do you have against kidnappers and blackmailers, terrorists and bank robbers? What about examples of violence and inhumanity? And so on.

Which of the following provocative topics particularly affects you and why: war(mongers), military (personnel), nuclear power (operators and supporters), tabloid newspapers, medical practitioners and/or medicynical doctors, entrepreneurs, big shots, bosses, bankers, speculators, politicians, rich people, billionaires, poor people, beggars, thieves, robbers, fraudsters, con artists, murderers, rapists, religious fanatics, hypocrites, men who abuse women and children, public clerks, civil servants, parasites, opportunists, turncoats, greedy pigs, smart aleks, money sharks...

Expand this list until it contains all those who you reject and who are repellent to you, and delete any who do not fit for you. If you are an entrepreneur yourself, you'll certainly want to delete this keyword, but you should nevertheless underline it, because the shadow of your own profession could provide particularly important and productive insights (see also the chapter "Choice of career" starting on page 226).

Practical Exercise

Part 1: Let the respective "anti-hero" appear before your inner eye and allow all your prejudices to rise against it. Then ask yourself: What would the world be like without people of this type? What would be missing in the world and for me personally?

Next, allow possible light sides of this character type to emerge. After this, complete the right column of the list with these newly-recognized light aspects.

Part 2: Put together a list of people from the past and the present who you find repulsive—anti-heros from Nero, Hitler and Stalin to Josef Mengele, Roland Freisler and Adolf Eichmann or Charles Manson and all of the characters that aggravate you personally. Play the same light shadow game with them on the intellectual level in your shadow diary.

Hopefully you will not find the same level of atrocities in yourself, but you could ask yourself, keeping the example of Hitler and Stalin in mind, if you were trying to advance a particular ideology, what part of you would push this forward and just how far would it be prepared to go? A character like Nero could help you to figure out just how far you might go to satisfy an ego trip. Using Josef Mengele, Nazi doctor and mass murderer, as an example, you could notice the extreme degree to which a part of you may be invested in the pursuit of research and science. The example of Roland Freisler, the Nazi judge, could show you clearly to what extent you might be willing to trample bodies underfoot to uphold a system you believed in. And Adolf Eichmann, the Holocaust accountant, could make you aware of to what degree a love of organization and bureaucracy could (mis)lead you. Charles Manson could be used to gauge where sectarian madness could propel you in the most extreme case. Incidentally, female monsters, whose names are infamous and known worldwide, are rare.

Reconciliation with the darkest Shadow

By now, I'm sure the list of negative characteristics that you've entrusted to your shadow diary has already grown. Here is another suggestion for dealing with the darkest shadow aspects.

Feel free to add any number of additional characteristics to this list and to delete anything that doesn't fit for you. The more you react to one of these words for a particular characteristic and its related provocative topics, the more likely it is to be one of your darkest shadows.

Using the example of *murderous*, which is likely to present one of the maximum challenges for most people, let's work through how you can deal with even the most horrible shadow characteristics and reverse their polarity. The normal standard questions that can help you with the other characteristics and that you definitely should use—for example: *When do I behave like this nowadays? Have I ever behaved like this before?*—will hopefully not help in this case. However, the following questions, which revolve around potential (future) scenarios, can open the gates to your own shadow realm: *Could I ever behave like this, and under what circumstances?* and *What would have to happen for me for me to be able to ...*

Practical Exercise

Think about which of these characteristics apply to you: selfish, egocentric, deceitful, untruthful, vulgar, bitchy, ugly, diabolical, shameless, weighed down, superficial, cold, dishonest, cowardly, insensitive, stupid, disgusting, masochistic, sadistic, resentful, hypocritical, know-it-all, quarrelsome, devious, condescending, jealous, greedy, stubborn, hot-tempered, spiteful, useless, backstabbing, fat, cruel, prone to gloating over the misfortune of others (i.e. schadenfroh), dirty, thieving, sick...

Reconciliation ritual: Find a friend who will say the characteristics of these and other negative lists out loud to your face. For this ritual, choose, above all, those characteristics that you suspect may be difficult for you to accept. The person you are doing this practical exercise with should wear a mask that hides their face. This is recommended, not only because this ritual is about working on your persona, or in other words, your own repertoire of masks, but also because it makes it easier for the other person to transition into an impersonal, anonymous state.

When the other person says the shadow characteristics out loud through the mask to your face, you will still feel affected, of course, but enough distance is maintained, because the other person does not mean it personally. The person thus says directly: "You are a liar". They then let this word take effect and repeat it until you can answer with "yes" because that "yes" has risen up from the depths of your soul. Should it take a long time for this to be the case, they simply repeat the reproach until you reach this point. In some cases, you will probably have to retry the characteristic once again at later time.

After your counterpart has confronted you with a certain quality, such as: "You are a know-it-all", let it take effect within you and then repeat very consciously, but from within: "Yes, I am a know-it-all. I can see that now." Repeat these two sentences again and again inwardly until you feel that they are right. Then say out loud: "Yes"! Repeat the sentences again loudly and add: "I can now accept that I am a know-it-all". You will probably even think of situations in which you have indeed reacted as a know-it-all.

Next, you can take a step back to the chapter "Gathering Gifts" (pages 152), and in a meditative state, release the positive gift from your know-it-all tendencies, for example, the gift of having a knowledge advantage, the passion for acquiring new information or whatever. Record your results in your shadow diary.

For instance: *Before someone were to murder my child, I could probably kill him instead ...* Or: *I could probably kill someone in self-defense ...*

The integration of even the darkest characteristics begins with insights of this sort. Accepting them is necessary because, as long as we don't manage to do that, the Law of Resonance will bring us into contact with people who represent this characteristic, and the more repressed the characteristic is in ourselves, the more dramatic such encounters will be.

Of course, your lists provide material for many reconciliation rituals of this kind. But keep in mind that less is more. Don't do too much all at once. It is better to go through a topic intensively and to have really felt it than to hurry over many things quickly.

When we meet the darkest and most frightening shadows within us, it usually takes some time before we can really uncover the gifts hidden within. Our fairy tale heroine Belle also has to live with her "beast" for a while before she becomes mature enough for salvation. Between insight and transformation, there will be a moment of shock, which is worth thinking about. Miller says in his book *The Golden Shadow*: "Nevertheless, it is of utmost importance that we do not totally identify with any of these negative, even evil dimensions that come into our awareness. To identify with shadow and act it out is dangerous and potentially destructive. Such behavior is completely different from our discussion of suffering a shadow insight (denying the temptation to act it out once it becomes conscious). We live with the tension between the old personality dimension and its newly discovered opposite until the new element is integrated into our conscious personality. We must bear the distress of owning this dark element until we find the way to incorporate it into our conscious self by using it in a creative and positive way."[30]

It is therefore by no means a matter of translating the dark sides and features into dark deeds and actions. Instead, it is about living on in the consciousness of their existence and of enduring this tension between the self-image that up to now had been filled exclusively with light and the darker image that has now been added. Immediately, a noticeable mildness towards those who show similar dark sides will start to set in. This will reduce the desire to condemn or objectify our judgment towards them. This feeling in itself will feel good and make life worth both living and loving.

Nevertheless, the truly decisive step only comes when we recognize the judgement-free energy in our own dark shadow aspect. Rape or abuse are terrible shadow aspects. As a perpetrator, it is difficult to see the pure energy of aggression within them. Those who discover the rapist in themselves will be shocked, and the shock may have a lasting effect. But it is possible via this path to find our way to our own strength, courage and decision-making ability. This step neither undoes our own deed, nor makes it any less terrible and must not lead to such crimes being repeated or even tolerated in general. The conscious or

30 Ibid Miller p.74

unconscious self-condemnation can, however, transition into acceptance of this sinister shadow, and this results in access to the energy blocked here. The situation can no longer be changed. Nevertheless, so that it does not repeat itself under any circumstances, this step into acceptance is extremely important for the perpetrator. There are more than enough terrible examples to prove that even draconian punishments do not protect against the repetitions of crimes. Acknowledgement and acceptance do protect against them and lead to a change of attitude that the Ancients called "metanoia"—deepest remorse.

Radium can cause cancer, but it can also be used to treat cancerous growths. Radium should therefore be seen in all its possibilities in order to really do it justice. Salt spices up the soup, but in large quantities, it becomes dangerous. With a knife you can both cut bread or kill someone. Poison can cause death, but can also be used to heal diseases. It is the transforming pure energy of the substance that needs to be seen in the sense of the words of Paracelsus that "the dose makes the poison".

You decide for yourself how much time your shadow and consequently your self-realization are worth to you. I can guarantee that everything that seems unpleasant at first will, over time, even start to be fun. To the extent that the gain in energy and joie de vivre becomes clear, your joy for life will increase.

In the long run, this therapeutic shadow journey will even turn out to be a large-scale project that serves to gain time. Nothing is responsible for as many absences as shadow—not only in the form of real absences as the result of illness and death, but also due to all the small absences that arise from daydreams, brooding and getting stuck in the unsolved and unresolved past, with all its unfinished and unprocessed business.

The mention of death in this context may seem frightening and exaggerated, but after more than thirty years as a doctor in a spiritual environment, I am convinced that overpowering shadow often conjures up death. A life comes to an end when its possibilities are exhausted, and it has fulfilled its purpose. People die in peace when they have learned what was to be learned for them in this incarnation. They die in stress when they don't even realize how they have long since stopped learning and their lives consequently no longer make sense. Modern people cling particularly vehemently to life, even in old age, because on the one hand, they hope to still learn something after all and take it with them, and on the other hand, because they have no idea what comes next. Both of these things are understandably frightening.

Every hour that flows into shadow work is therefore an ideal investment. The sooner the shadow work takes place in life, the better for each of us individually, but also for our environment and the whole world, and even for our life after death, when we join the circle of our inner images, both light and dark. This is the real background to the Christian purgatory myths. This after death situation is excellently portrayed in the film *What Dreams May Come*, with Robin Williams in the leading role, and accords well with my many years of reincarnation therapy experience.

Film Meditation

Watch the film *What Dreams May Come*. As the music of the closing credits starts to play, stay in trance-like state and simply close your outer eyes so that you can head off on the corresponding internal visual journey that now awaits you.

Once again, record your impressions in your shadow diary.

Inner riches and the diversity of life

Our light Shadow, our light potential

Sustainable work with the darkest shadow needs a counterbalance by turning to our unconscious light side. Both complement each other perfectly and each is reflected in the other. Take the time to also add to your positive list again and again. Naturally, the negative list can serve as a prompt. Which of the following good sides have already come to mind so far: beautiful, successful, elegant, buoyant, helpful, free, floating on air, creative, spontaneous, honorable, honest, courageous, visionary, strong, energetic, powerful, spiritual, sensitive, tactful, compassionate, uplifting, caring, loving, inspiring, heavenly, angelic, enlightening ... Hopefully the list of famous personalities from the past and the present with the positive qualities you admire will also contain several entries, for example: Mother Teresa, Albert Schweitzer, Nelson Mandela, Florence Nightingale, John Lennon, George Clooney ... In addition, there are all your personal heroes and heroines, who have touched your soul and who your soul has recognized. For me, they are, for example, Sister Alberta, Hermana Maria, my daughter Naomi ...

Practical Exercise

Deal with the heroes and heroines in the same way as with the anti-heroes. Find out what your personal relationship to them is and how what you admire in them wants to grow within you. Ask yourself: Where—in which particular aspect of my life? When—in which particular time or phase? and of course, how and to what extent?

Have the courage to work on another light figure in your shadow diary every now and then and to integrate the qualities that you admire in them into your own life.

In nature, the brighter the light casting it, the darker a concrete shadow appears. Does this also apply to people? The more positive or "holy" a person is, the more negative or unholy their shadow?

We know that Saint Paul, the political propagandist for Christianity, was previously the most notorious slaughterer of Christians as Saul. His transformation from Saul to Paul survives today in expressions, such as a "Pauline conversion" and the "Road to Damascus". Even in his later life as an apostle, Paul continued to talk of shadow experiences. In his letter to the Romans (Rome 7,15), he confessed: "For I do not understand my actions: I do not do what I want, but what I hate". Similarly, it is well known that the playboy Francesco transformed himself into Saint Francis of Assisi, while the beautiful Mary Magdalene transformed herself from whore to saint and Augustine from eloquent opportunist to mediator of the doctrine of salvation. But are we prepared to acknowledge the principle behind it: The brighter the light, the darker the shadow, and by analogy, the brighter a personality, the darker their shadow.

And, of course, the reversal of this also applies: the darker the shadow, the greater the potential for light. This is the reason why fiery love often ends up as cold hatred. This transformation can, but does not have to happen. If those involved keep a watchful eye on their shadow and each of them integrates it into their own life, this can even foster their love, because it makes both lives richer and more complete. It is all about awareness, transformation and metanoia, a true change of attitude. As Gitta Mallasz says: "Don't improve the bad. Strengthen the good,"[31]

In terms of shadow, this means that we actually need to be more careful with regard to a U.S. President Obama than with regard to his predecessor Bush. Obama drums up courage ("*Yes, we can*"), announces that good things are coming, as well as the transformation ("*Change*") needed to get there. We all love that, and as a result, he was immediately rewarded with the Nobel Peace Prize—but he has yet to earn it. One potential danger is that shadow will also strike him down, and he will, for example, start wars for good. But then again perhaps Fate will help him out instead. No sooner had he allowed oil drilling off U.S. coasts—contrary to his election campaign promises—one of the biggest oil disasters in U.S. history put this decision back into perspective.

The shadow of his predecessor George W. Bush was easy for most of us to see through. Bush lived out his dark shadows in a direct and thinly-veiled way by instigating wars under false pretences and undermining civil rights. Of course, he also tried to dress up such things in illustrious robes and propagated it as a crusade against evil. But only very naive people really fell for that, just as hardly anyone really "buys" the "holy war" of the radical Muslims fighting on the other side.

Bush lacked conscious awareness to an extent that was appalling for a man in his position of responsibility: right to the very end, he stood bewildered in the face of polarity and could not get a grip on his own shadow side. At no point did he understand why he would go down in history as the U.S. President who, through his actions, multiplied terrorism and spread it throughout the world. Not even the reality of the facts and figures

31 Mallasz, Gitta, *Talking with Angels*

Shadow diary

Where do I fight against my own problems using others? What do I not let anyone else get away with but myself? Where do I measure with double standards? Where am I suspiciously good, demonstratively upstanding and noble? What do I forbid myself and others from doing? Which people, especially historical figures, seem evil to me?

Please note down your realizations with regard to these questions in the shadow diary.

was able to disrupt the illusion of his perceptions. This is one of the great dangers of consistent shadow suppression: madness. William Miller writes: "What is distressing is the fact that those who most strongly deny their shadow potential are the very ones most likely to be overcome by it."[32] We were able to, and in fact, more or less had to expect such things from Bush. But everyone expects good things from Obama, and the danger is that his (unconscious) shadow may give rise to nasty surprises. Nevertheless, the hope remains that he is a self-aware person who is able to see his shadow side and thereby avoid its unredeemed manifestation with the help of this awareness.

In light of such realizations, many so-called "holy people" should have immense "holier-than-thou" shadows. On closer inspection, this is also the case. Since there can be no taboos in relation to the topic of shadows—taboos (in thinking) represent the biggest shadow traps—nothing is considered sacred in shadow analysis; quite the contrary, the sacred is seen as particularly suspicious. Thus, in the search for those who are truly holy and whole, not even the popes, the Catholic representatives of God on Earth, are spared. They are either truly whole and holy, as many faithful followers of Pope John XXIII assume,

32 Ibid Miller, pg 11

or particularly striking shadow representatives. Thought could be given to the moment in the life of the Polish Pope John Paul II when he threatened pharmacists with ex-communication if they—in the era of AIDS!—were to sell condoms.

Those who want to drive away evil but who nourish their ego while doing so are unlikely to be on the right path and probably won't come closer to salvation. But those who, on the path to salvation, increasingly expand their limited ego in the direction of shadow and who manage to integrate more and more aspects of themselves and of the world instead of excluding these, will reduce their shadow and come closer to wholeness and self-actualization.

Split personalities

In addition to the storefront and shop counter view of life or the house with twelve rooms that forms our shadow palace, there is a further model that also does justice to the shadow in an excellent way. It stems from the Psychosynthesis approach developed by the doctor and psychiatrist Robert Assagioli and is based on split personalities. Probably the most well-known example is the literary treatment of the theme in Robert Louis Stevenson's novella about Dr. Jekyll and Mr. Hyde. While Dr. Jekyll leads a respectable life during the day as a highly upstanding citizen, Mr. Hyde does the exact opposite at night. In the film *Belle de Jour*, Catherine Deneuve gives a ravishing portrayal of the middle-class wife Séverine, who does just the opposite. While she rejects her husband's sexual advances every morning, evening and night, in the afternoon, she is the tantalizing femme fatale for the special wishes of men who in the daytime allow their sexual shadows to dance for money. They demand things from this beautiful woman of the day that they would never dream of expecting from their middle-class wives. This beautiful woman fulfils their wishes with such devotion because she does it for herself, or more precisely, for one of her split personalities. Both Séverine and Dr. Jekyll offer their shadow side, which is scarcely able to be integrated into middle-class (stuffy) life, an outlet during the day, respectively at night. In this way, they keep their lives in balance—at least for a certain amount of time. If they did not live out these possibilities and could not allow their dark energies to run free, they would find living in the other light pole difficult to endure. The unlived, pent-up energies would put them under pressure. This may give us a hint as to how those who do not have such outlets, but do have corresponding needs, feel in their highly-respectable lives. In truth, we all have corresponding safety valves, but we are mostly unaware of them:

- In the dreams we have at night, and especially in those dreams that are filled with dark fear and horror, the so-called nightmares, corresponding energies are discharged. Every nightmare is a small bit of shadow therapy, whether we are aware of it or not. In this respect, we could be grateful for them.
- Our mistakes are also expressions of shadow, which can draw our attention to the dark energies in our spiritual depths. They therefore also deserve our thanks.
- Disease and other symptoms do their bit to express our repressed dark sides. We would simply have to approach them and learn to listen to them in the sense of *Disease as a Symbol*.
- What we don't like about our body could very easily draw our attention to where we're stuck and where we need to grow.[33]
- In the case of accidents and all kinds of other problems, from our relationships to our career, shadow energy also demands to be given opportunities to appear on the stage of our lives.

---

33 In this respect, see *Der Körper Als Spiegel der Seele (The Body as a Mirror of the Soul**)

The question is whether we pay attention to these attempts or whether we shove them back down through the trapdoor. If we do the latter, we will continue to offer our winning smile to the various audiences in our lives who view us favourably, and we will do this in the hope that they will believe what we want them to believe, namely that we really are what they see. Nevertheless, this can only work for a certain time—until the back-up of shadow energy grows so large that it produces another outburst that is less easily overlooked.

Basically, we can see the world with all its challenges as a teacher or as an enemy. The end result of both variants is completely different. Anyone who accepts "Mrs World," with all her dark aspects, as a teacher will in the end be taught well and will also often be taught a lesson, and perhaps even become wise. This student may not be good, but will certainly be relatively whole. Anyone who regards her as the enemy will end up surrounded by enemies. Possibly such a person will feel like a good human being, but will not actually be whole, and with their overpowering and threatening shadow and its corresponding resonance, they will bring wholly disastrous results. In accordance with the Law of Attraction, we get what we are in resonance with. If nothing else, we at least have the power to choose in this respect.

A further decisive point is whether we see ourselves as victims or instead recognize how, based on our own inner structure, we have brought ourselves into resonance with the respective events involved. This is also the difference between the immature experience of the child, who is at the mercy of events, and the developed experience of the mature adult, who both grasps and consciously accepts their own responsibility. The topic of resonance cannot be brought to mind often and deeply enough.[34]

Ultimately, it is always a waste of energy when we search for alternative causes as to why an event in our lives should not lie within our responsibility. The more primitive option is to seek the

34 In this respect, see *Die Schicksalsgesetze* (*The Laws of Fate**)

blame in someone other than ourselves. Basically, it is advisable to replace the word "blame" with "responsibility" and to not only always look for it within ourselves, but above all, to actually find it. Those who look for blame, of course, find it and, in the end, are surrounded by it on a large scale. Those who seek responsibility and recognize the blessing contained within it will find both, and in the end, will be blessed and grateful and hold responsible positions. The Bible tells us: "He who seeks shall find". In accordance with the Law of Resonance, we always find what we are looking for. We have the choice! The following poem Autobiography in Five Chapters[35] also emphasizes the value of patience along the path of shadow integration:

1)
I walk down the street.
There is a deep hole in the sidewalk
I fall in. I am lost... I am hopeless.
It isn't my fault .
It takes forever to find a way out.

2)
I walk down the same street.
There is a deep hole in the sidewalk.
I pretend I don't see it.
I fall in again. I can't believe I'm in the same place.
But it isn't my fault.
It still takes a long time to get out .

3)
I walk down the same street.
There is a deep hole in the sidewalk.
I see it is there.

35 http://www.freespiritualebooks.com/uploads/5/0/5/8/50589505/the-tibetan-book-of-living-and-dying.pdf

I still fall in ... it's a habit.
My eyes are open I know where I am.
It is my fault.
I get out immediately.

4)
I walk down the same street.
There is a deep hole in the sidewalk.
I walk around it.

5)
I walk down another street.

In the final analysis, everything that prevents us from enjoying a life, in which we are healthy, happy, satisfied and at peace with ourselves reveals itself to be shadow. In other words, if our life is not wonderful, shadow must be in play and be the cause of it. The Shadow Cabinet of Split Personalities is a particularly delightful level for getting into contact with our own shadow sides. Sometimes these sub-personalities can become so powerful that they acquire psychiatric relevance. But even where this is not (yet) the case, they are in the game and play a far from insignificant part in it. Usually they do not split off completely, but rather function as parts of our personality. In the course of our childhood, youth and later life, they were excluded because of the values and convictions that prevailed in our environment. Now and then, they are given—mostly unconsciously—some space, which they then discharge their energies into. They show up behaviour that we as a person(a) find unacceptable. This is why we push these parts to the outer fringes of our lives and only rarely and unintentionally allow them a more or less small window of time, which on top of everything is usually very embarrassing for us. However, if these parts of our personality have gained too much energy due to very long periods of suppression, and if they have bunkered this energy and want to carry things too far in releasing it , we sometimes firmly show them the door and really split them off. When this happens, we feel no personal connection to their behaviour, as in the example of Dr. Jekyll and Mr. Hyde. The two archetypal stories of *Autobiography in Five Chapters* , the beautiful woman of the day, and Mr. Hyde, the frightful man of the night, might inspire us to go in

Film Meditation

Depending on whether you feel a greater connection to split-off parts from the sexual domain or to those from the realm of aggression, watch the film *Belle de Jour* or one of the many film adaptations of Dr. Jekyll and Mr. Hyde. Do this in a conscious way as a kind of therapy session. As the music of the closing credits starts to play, close your eyes and let your own associations with the topic rise to the surface. Then entrust these to your shadow diary. Repeat this the next day with the film that was your second choice.

search of our what divisive elements might be sprouting up like mushrooms through our own personal cracks.

A colorful inner family

In order to further encourage you to consider your own split-off personality traits or sub-personalities before they multiply like mushrooms and push through the cracks in your life, I would like to tell you about my own personal "subtenants":

First of all, there is the *greedy Rüdi*, who even as a child, when asked to give his sister some of his chocolate, was quoted as saying: "Eating it yourself is more fun". Even today, Rüdi still has a lot of trouble not to bolt down his food, but to eat slowly instead. Fate took pity on him and sent him a foster daughter who eats so slowly that you could almost fall asleep while waiting for her to finish. Nowadays, he even has to write books on the subject. And, of course, he learns best about what he—as a fasting doctor—is teaching. But the greedy Rüdi is still sitting at the table. He has patiently sat out all sorts of tricks from no longer eating anything during a phase of Pranic nourishment to being a teacher for the process of readjustment to food after a period of fasting. In the meantime, he is like a snake: he can lie resting for days and then suddenly, when everyone least expects it, he pounces mercilessly on some poor paltry buffet.

The doctor in me is grateful to the greedy Rüdi for the connection that I have to nutrition and to my tendency to test out all sorts of fasting and different diets on my own body. Without him, I would not have tried out all manner of tricks in the field of nutritional science and would not have continually dug deeper, all the way into the terrain of biochemistry. Over thirty years of fasting seminars can be chalked up to his account, and in this respect, the little "greedy guts" has already indirectly helped many others to a great degree as well. For me personally, he has helped me to achieve the only figure that suits me, and, of course, he has already allowed the two of us to earn quite a lot of money as part of a double act.

Professor Wise Guy, also known as *Dr. Know-All* (cf. Brothers Grimm), lives just around the corner and also has his embarrassing sides. But since these are sufficiently well known, I will only deal with the gifts that this sub-personality provides me with. This part didn't split off, but instead has subordinated itself to the rest. The fun that this part has in knowing everything better and more accurately is something that the system as a whole can be thankful for. This has provided us with a lot of information and background knowledge that we have often been able to put to good use. When writing books and holding seminars, the professor is always present, and more often than not, is very helpful. The fact that this part of me, with his precocious manner and not uncommonly greater knowledge, caused the blood of many a teacher and his step-father to reach boiling point, can no longer be changed; it can merely be accepted and tolerated.

Playboy Roger liked to come back to school with a tan, even in winter, after he had skipped classes, supposedly due to "being indisposed". School typically didn't suit him very well. Upon return, he would provocatively smear a special brand of lip balm on his lips that was designed for skiers. This, in combination with his facial tan, had only one purpose in the classroom: to make perfectly clear where he had spent the past few days. Through all of this, he enjoyed getting on his teachers' nerves and entertained his classmates with fun ideas and small pranks because he was so bored with school. When he finally—relatively late—became interested in girls, things at least became easier for his teachers.

Incidentally, it was this part that also, of course, managed to keep the inner child alive for us. When it comes to being a bit sloppy and careless, he typically tries to sell this as a result of his playful instincts. In any case, this part learned to entertain others from an early age. The idea of the mandala colouring books and many of the games in his various seminars can be attributed to the pronounced drive of this part of me for playfulness and painting. This part was also was a great source of inspiration for courses like "The Senses, Sense and Sensuality" and played a decisive role in initiating my own sensual-erotic liberation. It was he who found the right teacher at an early age, who then helped us to progress in so many ways, not to mention the many fantasy figures who were helpful for us along the way. His fertile imagination may not always have been easy for the mother we shared, but it later contributed to allowing things to be done in a more left-field, laid-back and easier way.

In this respect, a book like *Floating: Enjoying the Lightness of Being** owes its existence to him and certainly also the idea of tracking down shadow in this book using jokes and humor. Of course, the book about the lightness of being didn't appeal to a mass audience, and the majority of people will not choose to hunt down their shadow using jokes. In our neck of the woods, we enjoy worrying and torturing ourselves far too much, but for some, their shadow has actually given them a lot of fun and great pleasure. And as Jacques Brel put it, why should we put so much effort into searching for the truth in coffee grounds, when it is so much more pleasurable and convenient to find it in wine?

The trampling *Rhino-Rüdi* remains a little loved sub-personality, who ensures he gets attention in a loud way, and who, after so many bestsellers, successes and stage appearances should have long since learned to tread a little more lightly. Nevertheless, apart from the potential trouble he causes, he has also brought many gifts. For example, he has contributed greatly to our general assertiveness, as well as initiating a lot along the opposite pole: from " treading quietly" in connection with mantras and Zen meditation to Kin-Hin, the conscious, attentive walking of Buddhism. The latter is an exercise specially developed for *Rhino-Rüdi*.

As an example for the late development of a shadow stowaway, it would not do to keep the *paranoid Rüdi* under wraps. Until my mid-thirties, I was relatively carefree about theft and did not lock doors. Then, during a sacrificial ritual in Nepal, my wallet, with all my documents, was stolen. At this point, I was still able to interpret this quite esoterically as an invitation to give more voluntarily and remained carefree. When, one night in Poona, literally everything was stolen from me except the mosquito net I had slept under, I cycled– without glasses –and with the mosquito net as a loincloth to the daily dynamic meditation the next morning, feeling quite unsettled. In my stomach, I was already sensing a new and quite astonishing rage against thieving Indians. But when, in my mid-fifties, the window of my car was smashed in front of the Bishop's Palace in downtown Augsburg in broad daylight and a lot of things were taken, in particular, my laptop with half of a book manuscript that had not been backed up, as well as many unpublished articles, the paranoid Rüdi was born. Until then I had been a follower of Epictetus, who as a Stoic, said that everything lost and stolen is to be regarded as returned. But, all of a sudden, my stoic serenity was gone, and I developed a kind of security obsession with regard to the laptop.

Shadow diary

Write the story of your own "sub-tenants" in your shadow diary, and bravely give them free reign to guide your hand—almost in the sense of automatic writing. Try not to make a big esoteric issue out of it; just get started and write down the first thought that stumbles across your mind. It's not about structure or legibility, grammar, spelling or syntax, but about the content of the present given in this moment. The sub-personalities have not been well brought up, but will want to participate immediately and to finally do their best (for everyone) to tell their part of your common story. Wait until the very end to read through everything. You might be surprised.

Of course, sub-personalities and shadow aspects that emerge so late in life can expect to be closely observed and are therefore easier to deal with. The gifts that this annoying sub-tenant has bestowed include advances in data protection and sympathy with the insurance and reinsurance specialists from the conservative, middle-class camp, which I have been far less inclined to make fun of ever since.

And this is only a small trial sample of the various sub-tenants who inhabit my soul. Also worth mentioning would be *Dr. Quick to Grumble* and the little *poisonous imp* that all my patients know only too well, because he digs his finger into every wound. In this regard, one of my employees said: "We do not do therapy; we are therapy".

Naturally, it is once again the case that the most unpleasant of our sub-tenants are the most important. The integration of their messages and qualities is most essential. Psychotherapy at the level of inner soul images with one's own sub-tenants is a good way to get to know and accept one's own shadows. Once they have been identified, the stowaways are more than willing to help and are very honest. They answer any question asked to them in the form of the first thought that springs to mind. It is simply necessary to catch this thought in time. In addition, they are sometimes quite funny and often very cooperative. They are merely concerned with knowing that the qualities that they express will continue to be represented in life.

Sub-personalities and relationships

When you enter into a relationship with a person, your respective sub-personalities also come into contact with each other. This is something that it is hard to consciously prevent. The respective sub-tenants and stowaways also develop a relationship with each other and have to learn to get along. What is particularly interesting in a partner relationship is the family circus that arises as a result.

As a rule, the bright sides have few problems with each other, because they typically already got to know and like each other at the very first party. In the early stages, they are happily put on show and placed in the centre of attention. In contrast, the stowaways in our respective life ships usually remain hidden for a long time, and at the very least, this is certainly the case during the initial phases. It is only after we begin living together that they start to gradually sneak in unasked and to get up to mischief in our everyday life.

When the *Princess on the Pea* plays together with the trampling *Rhino-Rüdi* at home, the charm of this duo often knows no bounds. However, when *Neat-Freak-Rita*, who is on a mission to make the whole world function like Switzerland in terms of hygiene and efficiency, and the not-yet-mentioned *casual-slob Rüdi*, who considers his own disorder and chaos to be a mark of creativity, cross swords, no washing machine remains dry. At this point, an extensive realm of shadow opens up, which can best be mastered using humour.

Shadow diary

Which sub-personalities have been stirred together in our relationship? What aspects stir things up and get us stirred up? How different are we and how impartial are we towards our sub-tenants? Which sub-personalities of my partner do I particularly like (least), and what does that tell me about my own shadow?

Please write down your answers in the shadow diary.

The more serious level for this can be found in our book *The Traces of the Soul. What our Hands and Feet Reveal about us*[*36].

As a matter of fact, when we *ask for someone else's hand* (in marriage), we would do well to ask ourselves what kind of hand we are actually dealing with. Our hands do not always fit equally well together by any means. The shadow of a relationship can also be foreseen in this particular aspect. Even after the fact, it is still fascinating to take a closer look at the hands that we have placed our fate in—and to closely study those feet with which traveling as a twosome through life has probably not been as easy as it seemed in the beginning when we simply naively wanted to *go out* together. In this respect, simple

36 In *Die Spuren der Seele: Was Hand, Fuß und Augen über uns verraten*

Meditation

Read Meditations 1 & 11 aloud to yourself and initiate an encounter with your partner and their sub-tenants. Meet at a party, consciously take time for each other and consciously get to know each other.

Then come back with a deep breath and record your impressions in your shadow diary.

forecasts regarding potential shadow realms open up, possibly even before these are excessively charged with spiritual energy.

Carnival of the Shadows

Mardi Gras and Carnival used to be traditional playgrounds for Shadow to run free, and as such, were good for our health. To a certain degree, they still have this playground function. For this reason, many find these events horrible, whereas for some they are source of great pleasure and joy. In effect, these periods can almost be interpreted as a form of protection against the unwanted outbreak of sub-personalities. Those who use this "fifth season of the year", as it is referred to in the Rhineland region, to allow some space to those aspects of their personality that are normally not given the chance to run free prevent these aspects from becoming suppressed and separated. If Séverine had let her hair down acting the part of the courtesan during Carnival, she could have spared herself her daily performance as *Belle de Jour*. Similarly, if Dr. Jekyll had cruised the streets more often as a fiend, robber and murderer during Carnival, he might have been able to take this load off the nights in his normal life. In this respect, playboys and playgirls, bank robbers and vagabonds, Zorros and cowgirls, heroic Indians and daredevil pirates may be much better off finding their place in the fifth season than during the other four. If you are a bank director and you act the pirate for yourself and your customers during Carnival, you will be less of a problem than if you do so behind the scenes and are secretively active all year round. Eventually your cover will be blown—as happened just recently—and this then usually leads to a great deal of resentment. The open declaration of it during Carnival, in contrast, tends to go down really well and the matching costume is viewed just as favourably—in fact, the wilder, the funnier. In this sense,

Shadow diary

Part 1: What did I like to go dressed up as to Carnival in the past or what do I still like to go dressed up as even nowadays? Which dress-up disguises were and still are tailor-made for me? Even if I won't admit to celebrating Carnival or no longer dare to attend nowadays, which dress-up disguise would I like to celebrate in? What would my costumes be, and what would my roles and issues be? Or have I become a victim of the Carnival shadow so that I now simply take part in an institutionalized ritual in one of the Carnival strongholds in ceremonially-fixed roles, without really allowing my shadow some space and the chance to run free?

Please record your thoughts.

Part 2: Where does my own Carnival take place? On dance floors or in the office or maybe even at home? Where could I give my different sides the chance to run free in the future? Where can I put my favourite dress-up disguises to good use? Where could I let which aspects of myself run riot and live it up?

Write down your thoughts and ideas without censoring them.

the original role of Carnival could be rediscovered and used for the benefit of the soul.

With their smoking colts, those who like to go dressed up as cowboys seem to be displaying aggression as a shadow topic on the surface, but behind the facade, as the (young-cow)boy, they also have a lot to do with the shadow of the small, dissatisfied mummy's boy. Those who go dressed up as pirates would obviously like to finally be the plunderer and simply take those treasures they desire and those they treasure when and how they please. If a woman poses as Marilyn Monroe, it seems certain that she would also like to be the center of attention and seduce the president live on TV as the cameras roll, assuming, of course, that he is at least as charismatic as JFK. The squaw is definitely looking for a noble Indian and the protection he could provide her with. Based on these examples, it can be very rewarding to interpret your own past costumes.

Vacation as an outlet for Shadow

Dropping out of our typical role during our vacation is natural, and is all the more therapeutic, depending on how entrenched our traditional role is during the remaining eleven months. In particular, those who are not even aware that they are playing a role are living dangerously with regard to the potential unexpected outbreak of threatening shadow. In this case, it would be much better to consciously take a "break from the Self" from time to time. Your normally way of acting ends up becoming exhausting in the long run, as certain shadow aspects will definitely not be allowed out to play in everyday life. Often, that's just as well, since we don't want our investment consultants, hairdressers, dentists or plastic surgeons allowing their adventurous risk-taking side to run loose at any time. Nevertheless, during their vacation, they each could give this part of themselves a

Shadow diary

To what extent do I already use my vacation as a vacation from the Self? How could I do this in the future? Where have I been so far, where have I never been? Where would I have to go? Where do I always want to go? Where not at all? What does that tell me? Where could a vacation become shadow therapy for me?

... and don't forget to take your shadow diary with you.

chance to run free without a second thought. When on vacation, it is possible to change roles, to dance to a different tune, to sound out the high notes and push these to extremes and to test setting the tone in a different way, for example, a notch higher, more beautiful, more luxurious, more adventurous, more daring, more cheeky, more glamorous, more revealing and sometimes even two or three of these. On the other hand, a notch simpler, more modest, more considerate and humbler could also provide an enticing shadow experience and encourage us to take a vacation in a monastery, ashram or to undertake a period of fasting.

Meditation

Read Meditations 1 & 12 aloud to yourself and take your time to calmly imagine your next dream vacation. Afterwards, come back to the present with a deep breath and then record your thoughts in your shadow diary.

Collective shadow

A system of healthcare? Or of disease creation?

Up to this point, there have been several mentions of the collective shadow that may encompass the unconscious issues of a particular group or society, a culture, a religious community, an institution or a profession. In a similar vein, the collective shadow of the healthcare industry has become particularly clear in recent times, and there have been many who have fallen victim to it. Instead of doing their best to promote good health, the relevant representatives in the pharmaceutical industry, but also health officials and even doctors, politicians and journalists have excelled at being creators of disease and the inventors of epidemics. The trick to all of this is extremely simple: dangers that are, in fact, always present are suddenly hyped up at any given time without (any real medical) cause or good reason and are then used for scaremongering purposes, as was the case, for example, with the so-called bird and swine flu. In such instances, entire occupational groups band together in a kind of shadow posse, thereby ruining their image and providing a prime example of collective shadow.

Working within the framework of early detection schemes, which are sold as "prevention measures", many conventional doctors also first recklessly spread the fear of cancer in order to then try to allay this fear with their own lucrative methods. It is in this use of non-existent precursors of cancer and exaggerated diagnoses to make patients more amenable to undergoing surgery that the deepest shadow of medicine is laid bare.

In addition, the German healthcare system has recently created a further terrible shadow, which up to this point has largely gone unnoticed. The billing of medical services is now linked to the severity of diagnoses. While this idea of giving doctors greater compensation for the treatment of more severe patterns of illness actually seems quite logical, it very quickly led many colleagues to make far more threatening diagnoses in order to "earn" more money. Nevertheless, diagnoses that are more severe trigger more fear and hopelessness. Anyone who sows doubt and fearful *second thoughts* when it comes to health is, however, instead summoning up desperate *second guessing* and clearly operating within the shadow domain. The Greek word *dia-gnosis* comes from *dia* (= through) and *gnosis* (= know, recognize). From a light shadow perspective, the idea here would be to look past the surface results in order to see through these to what is behind the symptoms. If we defy linguistic convention and shift the emphasis by only one letter, we end up with *di-agnosis*—double ignorance (*di* = two, *agnosis* = ignorance). Even though language experts would reject an interpretation of this type, in much the same way as they are consistently blind to the shadow, I refuse to believe that this is a mere coincidence.

It is definitely the case that individual words can help us in our search for shadow aspects, as for example, with the term "double-blind experiment". This term refers to the scientific requirement that, with respect to the self-healing powers of patients, both the effect of the psyche and the medicinal influence of the doctor need to be eliminated. At the same time, however, it blows the lid on an initial shadow aspect. Given that, in actual fact, most conventional doctors deny the existence of such forces, this naturally begs the question as to why they go to such great lengths to eliminate them in the first place. As such, the whole effort that is undertaken with double-blind experiments in itself actually becomes a kind of large-scale proof of the dual contribution of the mind to healing. Nevertheless, that is precisely what conventional doctors do not want to admit and this is where they chalk up their second shadow experience.

A far worse shadow reveals itself when we consider to what extent those conventional doctors who truly try to exclude these two decisive forces in their treatment, or in other words, those who transfer the scientific procedure to their practical work, are in fact operating "blindly" (in a double sense of the word). Naturally, all of this is done with the best of intentions, but still with catastrophic results. That is what is both tricky, as well as ingenious, when it comes to shadow. Thirty years of practical experience in the field of medicine have convinced me that fear and doubt make people sick and that causing them to feel panicked gets in the way of healing. In contrast, hope and faith heal, and there is little else that supports the process as effectively as a feeling of security and certainty. When it comes to health campaigns, it would therefore always be a good idea to check what is likely to come out if shadow aspects were also to be taken into account. A further shadow aspect of modern physicians becomes clear in the fact that they first force patients to be completely at the mercy of orthodox medicine only to then shift the entire (legal) responsibility back to the patient via their signature shortly before the operation. For one thing, it would be better to inform patients right from the start that they are always entirely responsible for themselves. At the same time, it would also be wise to only offer measures that are truly responsible in themselves, such as genuine prevention of the type suggested in *Disease as a Symbol*, instead of offering over-the-top early detection programs using methods that are often even more dangerous.

The alternative healthcare scene

Even the alternative healthcare scene has its own unspeakable areas of shadow, and in this respect, is also fundamentally flawed. When people are talked into believing that the way they are living is wrong and dangerous, it is the field of fear of illness and misfortune that gets cultivated, and by no means one of "contagious health". There is almost nothing in the area of nutrition that is not absolutely forbidden by one particular system while being praised to high heaven by another. In this respect, it becomes clear just how strongly shadow is dependent on the respective judgement involved.

There is one shadow tendency that is particularly obvious in the entire alternative medicine field. This is that almost everyone believes that his or her theory can explain and treat everything, if not outright heal it altogether. Something being one hundred percent the case in medicine is always false, and sure-fire promises of healing

Shadow diary

How do I react to grandiose healing promises? How great is my expectation that a miracle will happen? How much hope do I place in the latest, ever-changing methods in order to avoid dealing with the actual topic that I have long since been aware of? What state is my self-esteem in, and how overblown are my expectations?

How fanatically do I defend my particular way of life? Do I respect the uniqueness of every human being? Do I feel better because I am following a particular path? Or do I have a guilty conscience because I can't stick to any path?

Once again, write down your answers and thoughts in your shadow diary.

are forbidden with good reason. The various naturopathic treatments have actually gone astray in this respect and have correspondingly landed in a dead-end street that makes the shadow abundantly clear. Self over-estimation, megalomania, and above all, missionary-style fanaticism would be the ugly labels for this particular shadow. Its gifts are elevated self-esteem along with great dreams and projects, and the power to realize them.

Spiritual groups

Any group that has made enlightenment its aim automatically becomes susceptible to deep shadow in line with the motto: "Where there is a great deal of light, there is also a great deal of shadow." Whenever the ego is to be dissolved, it threatens to expand at the opposite pole and celebrate its triumph in an embarrassing way. As a result, oversized egos have become a kind of trademark of the spiritual scene. Quite a few of them consider themselves to be something better and accordingly present themselves in an arrogant and elitist way.

Anyone who wants to overcome polarity and thus our separation from unity, while at the same time constantly emphasizing their own singularity, obviously has a problem. Similarly, anyone who, in line with the dictum "My will be done", tries to get their own way in every situation and to constantly charge headfirst through every wall instead of accepting life with all its ups and downs is a victim of shadow—as is anyone who describes their own path as the only true path to salvation while at the same time promoting exclusion and the distancing of oneself from others. This, however, is the trademark of many sects.

Anyone who dreams of wholeness and deliverance, and then by means of positive thinking and affirmations expressly excludes the shadow, also has a shadow problem. Worse still, these people will actively encourage the creation of shadow despite their best intentions for achieving precisely the opposite.

Anyone whose meditation method claims sole validity clearly also has problems with the tenets of their own philosophy.

Shadow diary

How do my spiritual aspirations relate to my reality? What is my relationship to my ego? Do I really want to overcome it, or do I have spiritual projects that have been largely shaped by the ego?

Do I still fall for shadow traps and positive affirmations over and over again? Am I consequently on my way into tangled ensnarement instead of developmental unfolding?

Do I look down on "unspiritual" people? Do I missionize and if so, why? How susceptible am I to being spiritually led by others—as a victim? or as a perpetrator in the sense of "I know what is good for you"?

Confide your results to your shadow diary.

Watch out—Shadow! Tips for unearthing the hidden treasure

Slip-ups

The classic form of slip-up is the *slip of the tongue*, which transmits a message that is totally different to the one which was consciously intended. Our shadow and our personality suddenly and unexpectedly go their separate ways. A prime example is calling your partner by the wrong name in an emotionally-loaded situation, such as making love. This is a form of shadow outbreak that can hardly be more embarrassing. Any one of us, and particularly any guy, would desperately like to take it back, but that is not possible. The reality that has been unintentionally and unconsciously created now comes into play. Far more interesting than the strategy of denying and trying to sweep things under the carpet would be to ask the question of how this could have happened in the first place. Or better still, why this, in fact, needed to happen.

A patient of mine actually had this happen to him on his wedding night. Despite the fact that he and his partner had been together for many years, had already been blessed with a daughter and were in what would generally be considered a stable and happy relationship, she came close to breaking up with him on the spot. Forced by her to attend psychotherapy, he found the shadow topic behind the slip of the tongue. Although he had never expressed it openly, he was dissatisfied with the uptight and boring eroticism of their relationship. His slip-up in the form of this slip of the tongue—his unconscious awareness had chosen the name of a former girlfriend whom he had found far more erotic—finally brought the whole dilemma out into the open. His wife, who had already been the impetus for the therapy, eventually took over three quarters of the therapy hours and worked on her own corresponding issues. Two years and a four-week round of intensive psychotherapy after this highly-meaningful slip of the tongue, this shadow confrontation has brought both of them a huge step forward and made them much happier in their marriage, in which they are now also no strangers to fulfilling celebrations of lovemaking.

The alternative expression, the embarrassing one, which by means of the slip of the tongue, emerges from the shadows and forces its way to the surface ultimately carries the far more important message than the originally-intended "respectable" utterance. In the case of slips of the tongue, this alternative manages to outfox the super-ego, bypassing its control to break out of the shadow realm and into the conscious world. Such messages are unpleasant, but honest and meaningful. They have much more to tell us and a far more profound truth to voice out loud. In general, shadow utterances are always more important than those of the persona, our streamlined, well-ordered personality. In the short term, slips of the tongue are unpleasant, embarrassing and sometimes painful, but in the long term, they are beneficial for our development.

"Super-ego" is the Freudian term for that authority, which also filters our nightly dreams, making them seem alien to us, and which opposes our "Id", Freud's expression for shadow. The super-ego works to ensure prim and proper relations in the bourgeois sense, thereby creating shadow throughout life as the result of constant suppression. In this sense, the old master of psychotherapy at the same time already presented us with his own model for dealing with shadow. A prisoner of his era, he partly relied on its suppression, while at the same time also recognizing the opportunity that would emerge from its sublimation. Such sublimation would be aimed at finding a more agreeable level for the shadow energy involved. Without access to knowledge about the archetypes, however, any attempt to put this into effect would be largely doomed to failure, since energies cannot be shifted randomly all over the place, but instead can only be transformed within their particular archetypal environment. The energy of aggression contained in screaming fits of rage can, for example, be transformed into the courage to boldly push forward and face life head-on, but not for neatly organizing a writing desk. The former remains within the realm of aggressive energy, the latter points to the principle of reduction to the essential. In addition, the method of Freud's therapy was still highly intellectual and heavily influenced by the left-brain thinking and was thus strongly attached to the archetypal male pole.

Bursting into fits of hysterical laughter at a funeral is a further well-known embarrassing kind of slip-up. Even though the super-ego decrees that, for the sake of decency and all other good reasons, only sombre signs of mourning are to be shown, the hysterical opposite slips out in all its honesty. With embarrassing clarity, the shadow spontaneously makes itself heard in a *meaning*-ful way. In such cases, a mourning guest, or one of their sub-personalities, does not actually find the farewell sad, but instead decidedly amusing and perhaps even liberating. The analysis of such situations would quickly produce the corresponding shadow. In this kind of situation, the apologetic assertions or claims about how sorry one is for causing such embarrassment are not believed by anyone anyway. At a Catholic wake, this change of polarity from mourning to cheerfulness is actually even intended.

Action slips can be unconscious to a greater or lesser degree. "*My hand slipped*," says many a mother in the hope of being able to free herself from guilt in this way. Nevertheless, most of these slips are at least semi-conscious. With this in mind, a *slip* along your path that unexpectedly throws you off track and out of your usual rut already has a different quality to it. Whether it be classically on a banana peel in slapstick style, or a little more realistically, on an icy sidewalk, in such cases, you are not thrown off course without a deeper reason and goal. The analysis of where you land compared to your original destination is always valuable and infused with shadow. At the very least, every slip-up of this kind brings us firmly back to earth with a jolt.

Anyone who experiences taking a *misstep*—no matter on what level—can be sure of the shadow that has *stepped in* and come to light. No one *puts their best foot* forward accidentally, nor do they *get caught on the wrong foot* by chance. In the first case, the ego is directing the show, in the second, the shadow. Sometimes, in the latter case, we make a direct accusation to the devil. Those who say "To hell with it!" are right in wanting to send the mishap (back) to the devil and thus to the shadow realm. They could also talk about a slip-up "from hell", and in this way, point to the shadow as the origin of the mistake. Anyone who has been tripped up along their way has not been following their path in a completely straight-forward and upright manner. A small moment is enough to make this misalignment of the soul clear on the physical plane. In this way, we could use such small details in every moment of our everyday life to track down the shadow and wise up to its cunning tricks. When we "*cut off our nose to spite our face*" or "*shoot ourselves in the foot*", the matter is made clear linguistically. These expressions are synonyms for making an unwise move. Obviously, when dealing with dangerous topics, having a knife or gun in your hand poses a grave threat if there happens to be a slip-up.

Sometimes our slip-ups are not so much caused by the concrete mishandling of something but instead by the complexity of the subject matter. Testaments that intend only the best but end up achieving the worst tend to be the rule rather than the exception. Here the shadow shows up clearly in a multitude

> **Shadow diary**
>
> What slip-ups can I (regularly?) count on? In what ways have I slipped up in my life so far? What influence have such slips-ups had on my life up till now? Which of my slips of the tongue and action slips do I still remember particularly well? What do they tell me about myself in the here and now?
> Have I made a will at all, or is the subject of death still too hot for me to handle or too full of shadow?
>
> Make a note of your thoughts in your shadow diary.

of variations. Lawyers even speak of the so-called "slap in the face from the grave". By this, they mean a will that is hurtful and has a lasting unpleasant effect on those who are left behind. Often the pain is intentional, but far more often, it is an expression of unconscious shadow. The deceased wants the very best for the next generation, but nevertheless spoils everything for their children from the ground up, or more accurately, from the depths of their dark grave.[37]

Symptoms (of illness)

Every little slip-up is a symptom. Consequently, symptoms can be found on all levels of life and certainly not just in

37 In this regard, see Thomas Fritz: *Wie Sie Ihr Vermögen vernichten ohne es zu merken. (How you destroy your legacy without even noticing it)*. HDS, Weil im Schönbuch. 2007.

the domain of medicine. The word “sym-ptom” literally means “cut together”. When, at the end of filming, the final cut is made and the decisive ninety minutes are cut together from hundreds of hours of film material, the moment of truth arrives. Similarly, a symptom represents the final cut of a more comprehensive story, which then shows up in the symptomology in a condensed form. The small tick—the twitching of Bruce Willis's eyelid—in the highly-recommendable Disney film *The Kid*, which deals with the suppression of the inner child, makes this clear.

Many a time the overall composition of symptoms into a clinical “picture” has seemed to me to be like a work of art—a poetic composition of Fate that continually becomes more intense. By means of this “composition”, Fate starts *breathing down the neck* of the person concerned and even gets under their skin to help them make the leap towards tackling the upcoming shadow integration. By means of the symptom, a message that has otherwise been suppressed punches its way out and grabs our attention with a great deal of clout and intensity. The more willingly we show a symptom respect and acceptance, the less drastically it has to get mixed up in our life and mix it up. If we had paid attention to the issue involved straightaway, it would not have come to the symptomology in the first place. If we at least notice a symptom immediately, there is no need for a lengthy (medical) drama to develop from it, as this is nothing more than the creeping escalation of ignored shadow energies.

By making a list of the illness symptoms that we have experienced so far, and examining them in detail, we will amass an impressive array of our own shadow topics. If we translate these symptoms into the underlying tasks, as the process of disease pattern interpretation recommends, we will uncover an extensive program of work to be done.[38] This undertaking becomes

---

38 See *Disease as a Symbol* and *The Healing Power of Illness* (https://www.dahlke.at/international-editions) *or Frauen-Heil-Kunde, Aggression als Chance, Depression. Wege aus der dunklen Nacht der Seele, Krankheit als Sprache der Kinderseele, Verdauungsprobleme, Gewichtsprobleme.* (https://www.dahlke.at/buecherliste)

particularly productive when we combine it with the corresponding meditations and transpose the topic involved to the image world of our soul with the help of a guided meditation. If there is no special program for your own clinical picture, the meditation Self-healing is suitable for all issues, as it guides people to their own personal interpretation and processing. If your particular clinical picture is not interpreted in detail in any of my other books, it is very likely to be found in the reference work *Disease as a Symbol*.

Nevertheless, by taking a closer look, shadow manifestations can be recognized in symptoms on other levels, too. For example, road traffic accidents (quite apart from the legal questions concerning who is at fault) are always clear. However, all other accidents, even all the way up to the linguistic ones in the sense of slips of the tongue, are a public announcement of shadow. Utterances like: "That was the very last thing I wanted to say," "I can't believe I said that," or "I meant the exact opposite," make the faux pas, the "misstep," clear. In actual fact, I did say it or do it, and in doing so, I lent the shadow my voice or gave it a hand for one tiny honest moment. Slip-ups on all levels, be it when walking, acting and speaking, make us honest and lead us to shadow. In general, all of the aforementioned slip-ups in the sense of Freud's *Psychopathology of Everyday Life*[39] belong here and can hint at important clues. In the film just named, Disney's *The Kid*, it is merely the small twitch of the main actor's eyelid—a mixture of tic and habit—that the whole story of the shadow hangs upon. In the end, his inner child, who was pushed aside, or more accurately, down into the shadows in early childhood, is able to be integrated. The man as a whole has grown considerably, especially as far as his relationship is concerned. For that reason, the twitching has fallen by the (therapy) wayside.

---

39 Sigmund Freud: *Psychopathology of Everyday Life*. Forgetting, Slips of the Tongue, Bungled Actions, Superstitions and Errors

Since everything that is rejected can lead to shadow—in both senses of the word—this also naturally applies to those aspects of our body that we have rejected. My book *The Body as a Mirror of the Soul** is devoted to this topic. It uncovers, for example, the unwillingness to be *pushy* that has instead been pushed down into an oversized buttocks, the well-rounded attitude towards life that has slipped into a rounded belly or the shadow of goal-directedness that is clearly revealed in an duck-like, waddling gait. Naturally, we are not consciously aware of such signals, which is why they are lived out in the body. That a well-rounded belly reflects a suppressed longing for well-rounded perfection stands to reason. However, the same also applies to collective changes of form. The ever-expanding weight problem in modern industrial societies reveals to what extent carrying a lot of weight in society has slipped down into material levels.

Every conspicuous body-related symptom, from a bald head to a double chin, a flat bottom or bow-leggedness can be interpreted in its own right. Every aspect of form reveals content as well. The expansive body shapes bring the ancient ideal of the Venus of Willendorf back to life, but also reveal the collective shadow of the Great Goddess. Having long been persecuted by Christianity, she is now emerging from the shadow by the millions and making life harder to bear for the ladies in question in the truest sense of the expression.

But even the tiniest of our organism's signs can reliably help us to track down shadow. Fingerprints are not only of help for criminologists; we can also use them to recognize ourselves and our different sides. Our life-tasks are actually placed in our hands and written on our fingertips, but they are also found in the roots of our feet. The latter willingly tell us where we come from and what is still missing from our understanding of the world.[40]

40 In this regard, see *Die Spuren der Seele: Was Hand, Fuß und Augen über uns verraten (The Traces of the Soul: What our Hands and Feet Reveal about us*)*

Practical Exercise

Write the clinical pictures and symptoms of illness that have appeared in your life in your shadow diary and look for the corresponding interpretations. On a new sheet, place these opposite each in short form. Finally, find the similarities and look at the common golden thread.*

*In the future, the portal www.mymedworld.cc will offer an easy way to facilitate this process in many ways, as the computer will be able to filter and group together any accumulations of particular elements and archetypal principles, as well as more quickly identifying whether the symptoms refer more to the archetypal female left and lower body hemispheres or to the male right and upper body hemispheres and so on.

Film Meditation

For the benefit of your inner child, take a look at Disney's *The Kid*. Watch the lead actor's eye twitching throughout the movie and pay attention to when this symptom occurs and what it indicates. Close your eyes as the credits begin to roll, and on your inner screen, observe your relationship to your father, to your own inner child and to the opposite sex. How does your shadow make itself felt in all of this?

Confide your results to your shadow diary.

Bad habits, shortcomings

Over and over again, it is worthwhile closely examining our personal and collective *prejudices*, like a detective with a magnifying glass: prejudices about people of different nationalities, those with a different skin colour, those from a different social class, those with a different level of education, those with different religious beliefs, and so on.

In particular, wherever there is *envy*, there must also be shadow. Those who do not like people who flaunt their wealth are, when it all boils down to it, actually envious: a part of them is envious of the riches that the others have, and they would like to have this same wealth themselves. The envy shadow is very widespread and is linked to our addiction to money and possessions, which is one of the most dangerous addictions for our world. Behind it lies scarcity, or in other words, an unresolved emptiness. In archetypal terms, this becomes visible in the principle of reduction to the essentials, to which hard work, wise limitation, discipline and clarity belong—and which, at the same time, contain the solution for the problem of envy. The envious person can work hard and thereby fill their lack. Alternatively, they can learn to limit themselves to the essentials and to find clarity regarding their needs in order to wisely do without them.

Envy is also closely related to *sour grapes*. Those who begrudge someone something ultimately want it themselves. Envy and sour grapes therefore go hand in hand and are a plague of our modern times and society. But, of course, they also offer good opportunities to integrate shadow aspects and grow from these. Those who are able to perceive themselves as jealous and envious can see through this. They can either obtain whatever they are envious of by themselves or consciously choose to do without it, thereby recognizing how much dignity lies in a simple life, as, for example, Zen Buddhism teaches us. In both cases, they can more easily grant others what they themselves possess. In this way, envy and sour grapes act as fertilizers for development and neither of them will survive this exercise in consciousness.

Wherever *anger* comes to the surface, there is unresolved aggression behind it as a shadow. Those who projected their anger onto bankers during the financial crisis would actually have liked to have helped themselves to the pie and made a proper fortune as well; they are simply not consciously aware of this. Instead, the bankers get pilloried and punished on their behalf. Projecting all the way, we set ourselves up as the attorney for such vague entities as the "public interest" or "healthy common sentiment".

An even darker shadow feeling is cold *hatred*. Supposedly unforgivable injuries, injustices and rejections lead us down this dead end, in which one's own life can be completely ruined, and it is from such cold hatred that horrible deeds can grow. A hateful person has the features of this attitude to life written all over their face. The ill will that they cannot let go of ultimately leads to their own unhappiness and poisons their life. Giving up the self-hatred and the hatred of life that is linked to this hatred and then facing their own shadow would be the only way back to God, humanity and their own self.

A huge shadow is stuck like glue to the topic of *sexuality* in the conventional Christian world. Anything that is so rigorously degraded and repressed, while at the same time being so important—after all, the desire for sex is what keeps humankind going—must cast a huge shadow. Sure enough, the many millions of porn movies bought in a Christian country like Germany tell a clear (shadow) tale every year. Prostitution and pornography are shadow aspects of love that can be bought and sold and are the result of uptight Christian morality. This is precisely why they are so intensively fought against while at the same time regularly availed of by their distinguished representatives.

Once again, the Catholic Church makes this clear in a very drastic way. It sets itself and its priests the highest and loftiest goals, and it is for precisely that reason that the fall is then so dizzyingly deep. By forbidding sexual relations for priests, it attracts many people with sexual problems into its ranks. It goes without saying that someone who foresees only difficulties with sexuality will be fascinated by a sex-free vocation. Any young man in a rural environment who realizes that he likes men instead of women, or even little boys, will gladly flee into the protective framework of the church. The claim that there is no connection between celibacy and sexual abuse is as naive as the situation itself is sickening. The celibacy requirement that is equally as unnecessary as it is unchristian (in the sense that Christ has nothing to do with it) has the effect of downright luring in problem personalities. That these people cannot remain faithful to their good intentions in an environment that is hostile to sexuality is psychologically understandable. If an environment offers no natural ways to satisfy sexual urges, this will conjure up perverse practices. Where natural sex is already considered a serious offence, committing further serious offences won't really seem to matter. And so, paedophilia, blackmail, abuse and rape are added to the list. In keeping with shadow, it is hardly surprising that the church leaders themselves have also been guilty of veiling things in secrecy, brushing off concerns, looking the other way, glossing over crimes and ultimately even covering them up. This shows how repulsive this whole issue is to them. In this situation, we are witness to a lesson about abuse, its emergence and the attempt to conceal it, as well as the inevitable eruption of shadow. In the end, shadow always comes to light. Even the Catholic Church, the oldest and largest, or at any rate, most powerful corporation in the world, cannot prevent this despite its enormous cover up efforts.

What shocks so many people in such cases is the gulf between aspiration and reality. For those well versed in shadow aspects, this is hardly surprising. A religious community which has the audacity to reserve the highest and best offices for old men, because—in contrast to its founder Christ—it places everything that is masculine far above everything that is feminine, gives these old men, albeit unconsciously, the opportunity to abuse young boys. Or to put it another way, its members do not manage to protect these boys, who should actually be particularly dear to their hearts, from the sexual needs of many of the horny old men in their ranks. Whichever way you look at it, such shadow manifestations are always repulsive.

Those who are beside themselves with indignation about such incidents would need to ask themselves why they are reacting so violently. The answer is simple. In a society that is hostile towards sexuality, the shadow of abuse is huge. Many have been abused and have then later abused others themselves—often in a long chain that could be finally be broken by shadow therapy.

Of course, the Catholic Church is not alone with this problem. Wherever the aspirations are high and the people weak, there is the threat of shadow developments such as these. Consequently, it is hardly surprising that precisely the most renowned schools of progressive educational reform also found themselves swept into a similar whirlpool of abuse, rape and veiling everything in secrecy. Their original aspiration was to be particularly protective and nurturing of children as the weakest members of society. In practice, these children were then abused and raped behind the very walls that were adorned with such noble slogans.

Sexuality is the physical aspect of love and therefore also its shadow. Another shadow that is tied to love is overzealous *jealousy*. Rather than having your beloved partner's best interests in mind, you want to possess him or her instead. In this sense, jealousy is love that has plummeted down to the material level. Nowadays, this is considered more or less normal. In fact, a lack of jealousy comes close to being misinterpreted as a lack of love.

Money and any kind of *possessive thinking*—all the way through to fraud and betrayal—are also able to expose many shadows due to their commanding dominance of a person's whole life. Enriching oneself materially leads to shadow. Shadow work (shadow therapy), in contrast, means enriching one's Self. Those who do not truly possess their money are most probably possessed by it. In any case, we had already unmasked possessiveness as an essential shadow problem right from the very beginning. What we do not properly possess with our soul, ultimately often makes us possessed. If we truly possess money, we can become free of it in the spiritual sense and enjoy the possibilities that result from this. Or we can see through material possessions and avoid them as a dead-end street, perhaps consciously choosing to become a (begging) monk, for example. In between these two extremes, there is not a lot that allows our soul to remain calm and free.[41]

Shadow diary

What prejudices am I aware of? What prejudices can I own up to now, at this precise moment?

What experiences have I had with envy and sour grapes, as a victim and as a perpetrator? What role has greed played in my life?

Which fears determine my life? Have I already experienced feelings of hatred and revenge—and if so, when and where?

Are there feelings of inferiority and other complexes that I (still) allow to hinder me?

How freely can I deal with my sexual needs? How conspicuous is my reaction to the problems of others?

What shadows are attached to money for me?

Record all of the results of this self-exploration in your shadow diary.

In order to further shed light on the shadow, when making the negative list (see page 138), it is worthwhile going through any topics that rise to conscious awareness—from greed through to fears, from hatred through to feelings of inferiority—along with the corresponding complexes and delusions.

41 Read more in *The Psychology of Money** (See Bibliograpy)

Once something has been recognized as a source of shadow, it can also be of use for our own development and enrich and expand our life.

Bad-mouthing, self-criticism

Another simple way to get close to our own shadow is to note and consider noteworthy everything that others say about us, especially if said with critical and even mean intentions (see also the topic Bullying, page 79).

If someone wants to hurt us, experience has shown that the best way to do this is to shove a shadow in our face that is often easily recognizable from the outside. Something like this makes us angry very quickly and hurts us most deeply. The more wounded we are, the more shadow is in play—and the more grateful we could be.

The moment strong emotions are triggered, it is clear that there is an element of truth here. The moment we start to defend ourselves and lose our temper, the reproach must contain at least some grain of truth at its core that is important for us personally. The more angry and hurt our reaction, the more important the reproach or assertion is for us. No matter what our partner, our children, our business friends and competitors, and above all, our enemies say about us, we merely need to note it and consider it noteworthy. We should in fact already be grateful for this opportunity in and of itself. They are always right, even though they usually do not strike at the right level, i.e. the level corresponding to reality and truth. On the contrary, enemies tend to deliberately choose a particularly primitive and drastic level so that it will be hurtful. Now that we know this, however, they can no longer upset us so easily, but instead help us in a lasting way.

In this way, bad-mouthing transforms into opportunity. The moment they really strike home with us and trigger emotional reactions, this no longer counts as bad-mouthing, because now their assertions at least have a grain of truth at their core. For this reason, if we have declared enemies, who are constantly on the attack with us, this actually puts us in a good position in our search for shadow. Willingly, without pay and with full commitment, such enemies will constantly provide us with a supply of shadow aspects and highlight these clearly. We can hardly expect this kind of service from friends; instead, the latter are considerate, tactful and respectful. This is exactly what gets in the way of real help on the path to our own shadow and its integration.

So, when searching for shadow, be neither tactful nor respectful with yourself, and certainly not considerate; on the contrary, do without all three of these. Tact, respect and consideration are imperative in conventional society, but in the search for shadow, they always, and on the path of development, often get in the way. It is best to become your own worst enemy when searching for shadow and to shower yourself with every conceivable reproach. You—like your enemies in the external world—will be right on some level, and this is what you need to discover.

To keep this exercise in balance, you should then shower yourself with all sorts of honest accolades and compliments. Here as well, you can also exaggerate, and you will be right in essence. You should never forget this last point. If you do find yourself forgetting it, go searching in the shadow for the aspects of self-respect and recognition of your own person and your achievements that have been repressed. By the way, the process of self-reproach that is being suggested here is not nearly as unusual or difficult as it may seem at first glance. Most people are continually criticizing themselves anyway; they simply do it in unproductive and even dangerous ways. For women, this usually begins in the morning in their personal torture chamber, i.e. the bathroom in front of the mirror and on the scales. Anyone who calls out to or disturbs her during this morning self-criticism ritual will experience the whole, and at this point still unmade-up truth: "I'll be right there, I'm just finishing myself off." That is in effect truly what they are doing.

Many also finish themselves off during the rest of the day with constant self-criticisms. This hampers progress and does not bring them closer to reconciliation with the shadow. Instead, it leads to a counterproductive field of consciousness.[42] Admittedly, it is extremely effective in terms of reducing our self-esteem and dragging down our mood, but because it is not meant seriously and honestly, it does not lead to any recognition of the shadow. That this is the case can be proven very easily by simply agreeing to one of their self-critical statements of this type. If someone says: "Gosh, I look terrible today!", we are not allowed to confirm this under any circumstances, because otherwise the other person will get really angry.

The capacity for self-criticism is therefore very familiar to us. It is simply important to consciously note it and to consider it noteworthy. In our own case, it should be made use of straightaway in a therapeutic capacity. If we stick to the issue in question, we will quickly become familiar with previously-hidden aspects of shadow and will then be able to be finished with them.

If you criticise yourself for your clumsiness, you are addressing your inner butterfingers, the part of you with two left hands, who makes so many mistakes. This part of you is, of course, a shadow figure, just waiting for reconciliation and recognition so that it can help you to do things in a relaxed and easy way using solutions that come out of left field and that don't take things too seriously.

Those who bad-mouth themselves as *ugly* are thus speaking to that part of themselves which is out of harmony and that they have split off and chased into the shadows. Given that it is such a widespread attitude, it is reasonable to suspect that many people have this kind of ugly part within themselves. In any case, most of us are not in complete agreement with the

---

42 See in this respect *Das Bewusstseinsfeld CD (The Field of Consciousness* CD)*

body that we inherited from our parents or that we were given as a gift from God or Creation. In this respect, it is angelic harmony and beauty of the kind perceived in experiences of unity that are lying in shadow. Most probably we haven't cared for and trained this body properly because we weren't able to fight against our inner demons, or as they are referred to in German, our inner "boarhound". This mythical creature of the shadow realm mirrors our own sluggishness, desire for comfort and lack of regard for ourselves back to us. Naturally, we typically don't want to know anything about all of this and straightaway we land back in shadow. In this sense, taking our (inner boar-) hound for a walk is to be recommended to anyone who is on the trail of shadow. Lurking behind lazy complacency, it is structure and discipline that lie in shadow. These could facilitate spiritual practices, such as conscious fasting and spiritual exercises.

The most heavy-handed medical variant of repression and self-denial, and consequently then of further shadow production, is the attempt to have whatever is considered ugly simply cut off and away by means of so-called "aesthetic" surgery. This generates a lot of ugliness in and of itself, as well as an even greater loss of functionality and thus shadow—especially when trying to cut it out of the world.

Meditation

Read Meditations 1 & 13 aloud to yourself, then record your impressions in your shadow diary.

Afterwards, make yourself correspondingly similar over-the-top compliments, and from the first thoughts that come to mind, notice what you are most pleased by. After this, write any new insights on your negative and positive lists in your shadow diary.

Practical Exercise

What kind of self-directed insults and put-downs are you already familiar with? Go through your morning ritual in the bathroom in your mind's eye, for example, and take a look at what you beat yourself over the head with...

What bad-mouthing from others have you already experienced and what does it tell you about your shadow? If you really bad-mouth yourself as your own worst enemy correctly and somewhat exaggeratedly, what hits home the hardest?

Criticism, reproaches, advice

Often criticisms and reproaches, especially those from parents, are genuinely well meant. Parents love their children and simply want the best for them. They want their children to follow not only their advice, but also the same path that has worked in their own lives to some degree or other. Instead of fighting against this and building up resistance to it, we could thank our parents for their love and for wanting the best for us. It could also be affectionately added that their way—no matter how much we appreciate them as parents—is out of the question for us because we want to follow our own.

Ultimately, of course, everyone must go their own way, and so this way of dealing with parental concern should be generalized to a large extent and applied to all well-meaning people who have the best of intentions. Advice should always be treated with a great deal of caution and has the potential to lead us down completely the wrong path, because it is not fitting for us personally. A well-meant nugget of advice can end up strongly impacting many people and perhaps even crushing them altogether.

At the same time, criticism and reproaches are always valuable on the path towards shadow integration. These can never be so distant and far enough from reality as not to contain a grain of truth—even more so when they hit home or even deeply upset us. As soon as criticism triggers strong emotions, the same applies as to bad-mouthing. It would not be able to upset us so much if it was not true. Therefore, it is important to find the level on which it hits home, to take criticism seriously and to recognize it as an invitation for a confrontation with our shadow.

Shadow diary

What upsetting criticism can I now look at in a new way from this perspective and make use of for my shadow search? What words of advice, which used to get on my nerves, can I now recognize as highly impactful help for exactly this reason?

Write down your realizations in your shadow diary.

Resistance and defense mechanisms

By now, we should be well aware that anything we don't like, anything that doesn't suit us, anything that summons up resistance within us is an indication of shadow, and thus at the same time an opportunity for learning and growth. Wherever I sense resistance, I can be sure of running into my own shadow following up behind it. A huge field of shadow manifestations opens up here. Thorwald Dethlefsen wrote in *The Challenge of Fate:* "The greater part of human suffering arises from our own opposition to the circumstances of manifest reality. All things are in themselves of neutral merit. It is only our attitude which creates out of them the contrasting categories of joy or suffering."[43]

Loving what is:[44] Byron Katie, the American author, sums this up in her book of the same name. Shadow shows up clearly when we reject what is, and thus enter into resistance with reality. Resistance with what is always betrays shadow. As soon as resistance comes to the surface, shadow is in play. Tell-tale thoughts in this direction are: "That cannot be true", "This (life) is unjust", "It is unfair", "I don't like that", "I don't want to experience that", "God shouldn't allow something like that". When it comes down to it, all of these utterances, and not just the final one, amount to a kind of blasphemy against God. In effect, they are criticizing God's Creation and making their own suggestions for improvement.

In actual fact, everything can be judged just as easily in one direction or the other. The judgement does not lie in the things themselves or in the circumstances, but in the people making the judgement, who take one side, and in doing so, turn against the other. What finds approval in one place will reap rejection elsewhere and vice versa. Jennifer Lopez's curvy buttocks, when rhythmically moved, have been known to send millions of men into ecstatic frenzy. She is said to have insured each of her butt cheeks for a million dollars and thus truly seems to place a lot of value on her precious posterior. For millions of women and girls worldwide, however, very similar buttocks of corresponding proportions are a source of deep despair. They are appalled at themselves, or more precisely, at a precious posterior, which for them is worthy of nothing more than complaints and self-abuse.

Of course, in capitalist societies, possession is considered the most sublime of all feelings, but a wandering monk who lives from begging for alms does not feel the same way. Many people are more inclined to think that love is the most sublime of

---

43 Thorwald Dethlefsen: *The Challenge of Fate,* Coventure Ltd; 1st English edition, 1984

44 Byron Katie. *Loving What Is: Four Questions that can Change Your Life*. Random House: UK,

all feelings, but here again, there are others who may feel very differently about that because it has left them infected with a lifelong disease. Silence is the highest goal of many meditators, but as part of the torture of solitary confinement, it can drive people crazy. The followers of Eastern meditation strive for freedom of thought, but as part of their final year examinations, students hate precisely this phenomenon. Murder is a terrible thing, but the timely murder of Hitler or Stalin would have been a blessing for many and ultimately for the world. This chain can be continued indefinitely and probably finds its most beautiful form in the figure of Khidr, who is described in the 18th Sura of the Koran and interpreted by C. G. Jung. For Muslims, Khidr is a messianic figure and the first angel on the throne of Allah, who is responsible for sudden turns from happiness to misfortune and vice versa. When Moses asks Khidr to accompany him, Khidr cautions him against it, because he feels it will only lead to misunderstandings, but in the end, he goes with him, and straightaway, there is trouble after all. Khidr pierces holes in the fishing boats of one village so that they sink, kills a young, beautiful man and causes the walls of a city to collapse, which is then left defenceless. Moses is at first horrified until Khidr explains to him that he saved the boats of the village from pirates, who were on their way to steal them. He had saved the young man's soul, because otherwise he would have committed murder, and under the collapsed walls of the city, the poor inhabitants would find a valuable treasure.[45]

This chain of polarity reversals should not be misunderstood as the attempt to relativize or even legitimize inhuman or despotic behavior. A strict distinction must be made between a reality that has already come to pass and a potential future. Trying to derive the justification for unethical behaviour from this is a waste of time. However, if something has already occurred, even something that is atrocious, resistance to it usually leads merely

---

45 From: Marie-Luise von Franz: *Shadow and Evil in Fairy Tales.* Shambhala 2017

to suppression and thus to the creation of shadow. It would be far better to confront reality as it is.

Of course, in keeping with the same logic, resistance also has another side to it as well, as is the case with everything in polarity. In a dictatorship, resistance may be the only legitimate reaction, and as such, may then be fully justified. The Résistance—a coalition of the braver souls in France against the Nazis—later contributed to establishing a common sense of identity for the new France. Even under dictatorships, however, acknowledging the existing harsh and brutal reality is usually the best life insurance policy for resistance fighters and is certainly one that they would be advised to take out.

The Ego defines itself through separation and boundaries and the resistance associated with these. As such, it has to create shadow if it is to exist at all. As a result, if all resistance is given up, and all such boundaries fall away, the Ego will disappear without replacement. Those who no longer need separation and boundaries, who have found unity in themselves and everywhere else, are free of resistance and of their Ego. Their Ego has become one with the shadow. Both have entered the Self together. From this, it follows that anyone who sets off along the path of shedding light on their shadow is ultimately undertaking an attack on their Ego. This attack, which has the potential to be life-threatening for the Ego, can, by liberating shadow and Ego, eventually enable everything to flow together into the greatest liberation of all. All resistance is then given up and transformed in unanimity with all of Creation. Of course, resistance against the Ego is still also resistance. So in the end, we must give up this resistance as well in order to become completely free (of shadow).

Meditation

Read Meditations 1 & 14 and then take enough time afterwards to let the meditation continue to take effect and come to a satisfying end. After this, come back to here and now with a deep breath, and once again, record your impressions in your shadow diary.

The world of dreams

Dreams contain both types of shadow—wistful dreams, the positive shadow; nightmares, the negative. With respect to the dark shadow, William Miller writes: "When shadow appears in our dreams it appears as a figure of the same sex as ourselves. In the dream we react to it in fear, dislike, or disgust, or as we would react to someone inferior to ourselves—a lesser kind of being."[46] Even in our dreams, we try to avoid these kinds of shadow figures; often, we flee from them and feel stalked by them, as in nightmares of being chased.

The tendency to avoid shadow during the night, as well as during the day, leads to a build-up here as well, only to break out in our nightmares with a vengeance, as a way of gaining some space and our attention (respect) with a great deal of impact. Afterwards, some people still feel downcast and have the feeling that they have not yet shaken off the gremlins after they have woken up. Others, to the extent that they have really managed to leave the gremlins behind them, feel the relief that such a shadow therapy of this type brings with it. When it comes to the interpretation of the dream, the feeling that it leaves behind is especially important, even though we usually focus more on

---

46 William A. Miller, *Your Golden Shadow: Discovering and Fulfilling Your Undeveloped Self*. HarperCollins, 1992, pg 61

the symbols it contains. This is because we can still grasp these intellectually and see through them to a certain degree.

We have already noted that the language of the soul is a language of imagery. Even if we do not consciously pay any attention to aspects that are connected with our soul, this happens every night unconsciously in our dreams, regardless of whether we remember them or not. In the dark shadow of the night, we encounter everything that we have shoved down into our inner garbage dump: Wishes, longings, unprocessed feelings, fears, and life themes that have been long since forgotten, but are still unresolved. Everything that we do not expose to the light of consciousness returns in our dream world. In this way, our soul tries to make itself heard again and again. That is why dreams are among the most helpful and important instruments of shadow work. "Like an X-ray, or perhaps more aptly, like a portrait by a great master, it reveals a multileveled message about the dreamer's current psychic situation seen from a hitherto unknown or unconscious perspective," says the Jungian Edward Whitmont.[47]

The intensity of the feeling that remains after a dream is, as it were, a gauge of the extent to which shadow, or in other words, unconscious aspects, have been revealed in the dream. This becomes particularly clear in dreams during significant life crises, in which new, hitherto unconscious possibilities that were buried in the shadows force their way into our life. Archetypal dream elements during such times are often associated with strong feelings of fear, which are longing to be confronted. Various dark shadow themes that appear in commonly-experienced nightmares go hand in hand with these significant themes in life.

- Nightmares of being chased, for example, point to something that has been banished to the fringes emotionally, but which now wants to be taken notice of at all costs. For that reason, it downright stalks us without relent. After nightmares of

---

47 Edward Whitmont/Sylvia Brinton Perera: *Dreams, A Portal to the Source*. Routledge, London 1992, Ch 6, pg ??

this type, we should ask ourselves what we are running away from in life and what our pursuer stands for. Who or what does he/she/it symbolize?

- Nightmares about sitting exams, which usually end in failure, express low self-esteem and the fear of not being enough, of not being able to prove oneself. In any event, they confront the person concerned with fear, weakness and the feeling of being unable to succeed (in life). They may also point to something that has not been properly settled, to old scores or other unfinished business that we are still dragging around with us. It then becomes interesting to look at which test, in particular, has not been passed. This betrays where exactly something has remained outstanding. When it comes to driving tests, failing the test could indicate fears related to taking the wheel and steering one's "life car" oneself. Failing a mathematics test, could, in addition to suggesting problems with calculating in general, also point to problems with handling money.
- Dreams about falling also often arouse shock and fear. Humankind's original "Fall from Grace" in and of itself helps us to close in on the primeval human fear that is looming here. Falling deep is a synonym for losing practically everything except the chance for spiritual salvation with no safety net to catch us. It is a plunge into a bottomless, dark state of uncertainty. And yet the challenge of this dream topic is to let ourselves fall, surrender ourselves completely to the flow of life, give up all control, take more risks and develop more trust.
- Nightmares of being naked also signal suppressed shadow aspects, for example, when the dreamer finds themself as the only person without clothes in the middle of a public place. Feelings of embarrassment, shame and vulnerability characterize such situations. We would love nothing better than to become invisible or sink into the ground. The challenge in these kinds of dreams lies in summoning up the courage to show ourselves exactly as we are. How, where and in what form this should happen is symbolically revealed by which people the dreamer bares their all to.

- Dreams of water and floods indicate how deeply the water of our own soul wishes to to get back in flow and, if need be, to even overflow the banks and burst through the constructed walls of our own (emotional) dam.
- Destructive fire in dreams is often demanding radical cleansing processes, from which—like the phoenix from the ashes—it would be possible to rise again completely renewed.
- Dreams of loss indicate a long overdue need to let go of something, so that from a loss, a new lust for life can grow. The same applies to dreams involving something being sacrificed, or those about the disintegration of buildings or nature, or in extreme cases, about (natural) catastrophes.
- In periods of shadow in our lives, dreams of being torn into pieces can also emerge, an ancient mythological theme that many gods (such as the Egyptian god Osiris) fall victim to. In such cases, an old form is symbolically taken apart, thereby completely disintegrating, in order to arise again in a newer and more complete form.
- Dreams of flying usually convey the call to break out into further and freer areas of life. Nevertheless, they could also be giving the hint that a person is continually trying to escape from a situation, and is, as a result, refusing to deal with the demands of real life.
- Dreams about accidents call the well-worn grooves of our course through life into question and suggest that our old, familiar rut needs to be left voluntarily before we are forcibly thrown out of it in a painful way. Often, it is a question of discovering and following new paths that are out of the ordinary. The more comprehensive the changes demanded by Fate, the more drastic the accident will be.
- Dreams of paralysis or being frozen with fear are self-explanatory. Here it is necessary to ask yourself what is paralysing you: which fears, forms of resistance and blockades are causing you to freeze up and are preventing you from living your life, spreading your wings, getting your feet wet, taking roots and so on.

- If you get lost in your dream, can't find the right way (out) or are disoriented, you may feel panic. The lack of a way out of the situation provides the interpretation in itself. Generally speaking, the overview has been lost. If it happens in large buildings, it is the overview within ourselves, or if we lose sight of the right track, it is the overview outside of ourselves. The way out of such tight squeezes usually opens up if we are both willing and able to trust following unknown paths and are capable of re-orienting ourselves in life. Panic sometimes calls for a confrontation with Pan, the ancient god of nature, who was a symbol of polarity, and in keeping with this, with both sides of our own nature.
- A similar dream theme during times of shadow confrontation is revealed in just missing something, for example, when we continually just miss the train. Such situations convey a feeling of being lost, abandoned and forgotten. They can express how the fear of making mistakes has led to many missed opportunities in our life. Naturally, this begs the question as to what reasons keep us from being in the right place at the right time. Answers can be found in both the dream world and the real world. Perhaps we are carrying around too much baggage—in whatever form—which is slowing us down.
- In a similar vein, there are also dreams in which the dreamer admittedly keeps on running and running, but nevertheless, fails to get anywhere. Such experiences suggest an energy contribution that may not be appropriate for the current life situation of the dreamer. This running-on-the-spot, in what is typically a very frantic fashion, is self-explanatory. Fixed ideas about where exactly the path is leading to and just how to get there can lead to this desperation-filled dream experience with no hope of success. This begs the question as to whether taking a step back or to one side might re-introduce real and meaningful movement into their life once again.
- If the dream is about aggression, violence or rape, there is strong reason to suspect that these topics, which, in redeemed form, correspond to vitality, have been pushed into the shadows.

Important questions that arise from this are how to deal with this energy, and whether the dreamer is able to fight for their own objectives, to be assertive or to put up a fight if necessary.

- Dreams involving animals aim to re-connect us with our "animalistic side" and the corresponding instincts related to it. As such, they reveal our attitude towards our animalistic drives in general. In connection with this, one of the most frequently appearing animals in dreams is the snake. In the case of a poisonous snake, it is a symbol of primeval fear. However, it can just as easily be the evil serpent and the seductress who lures us out of the paradise of an ideal world. At the same time, the snake is the symbol of wisdom, transformation (in the shedding of its skin) and healing. In any case, it indicates upcoming tasks, such as renewal and the acceptance of polarity, and in this way, its poison becomes a remedy.

Shadow diary

Do I even remember my dreams, or do I lack this access to the inner world of my soul and its imagery? And has this access sunk completely into the shadow realm? Do I feel like unearthing this essential treasure of soul imagery and raising it from the shadow realm with the help of guided meditations? Am I prepared to restructure my nights and my sleep patterns in order to gain more access to it and my shadow aspects once again?

Are there particular shadow topics that recur frequently in my dreams? What might these be trying to tell me?

This list of common themes in dreams could be continued ad infinitum. Anything existing that in the language of the soul is pictorial in nature can express soul-related reality in a dream. Pictures and symbols never have just one clear meaning, but instead are ambiguous, thereby allowing multiple interpretations. In order to do justice to this richness of meaning and to identify

Practical Exercise

1: For one whole day, consciously capture all your daydreams and fantasies and record them in your shadow diary. As far as possible, try to uncover the major themes that recur frequently, both those related to light shadow and dark shadow.

2: Begin to take note of your nightly dreams and to consider them noteworthy. Address the major recurring themes of these as well with regard to both the light and dark shadow.

their significance for the inner world of the soul of each individual, it is therefore essential to recognize the feelings and sensations that are associated with them as signposts. In general, everything that we encounter in dreams in the form of pictures, figures and situations, is part of our unconscious soul landscape and thus also of our shadow landscape.[48]

Fantasies, daydreams

Although we are usually unwilling to admit it to ourselves, we spend an enormous amount of time in daydreams and corresponding fantasies. What comes to mind first and foremost in this respect are all of those thoughts and visions that we do not allow ourselves to entertain consciously, that in actual fact, we do not even dare to dream about at all, which is why they (must) sneak in via such channels. If we turn the tables and voluntarily devote our attention to this poorly-accepted dark realm by using guided meditations, this helps the soul as a whole, and

48 See *Schlaf—die bessere Hälfte des Lebens (Sleep—the Better Half of Life*)*

our access to the shadows of the night becomes easier with time.

Naturally, everyone has their own individual daydream topics, but here as well, there are also typical and archetypal patterns which are line with the collective shadow. Fantasies ranging from sexual desires to orgies and experiences that are taboo within a particular cultural context often play a role, as do fantasies involving abuse, or the exercise of power and violence, or a mixture of all of these. Whatever is regarded as perverted can make itself heard and grab our attention through our dreams at night and our fantasies during the day. Fantasies that invoke fear and panic also occur frequently and are cultivated (semi-) consciously through constant repetition.

In addition to the negative shadows, we also work on many positive shadows in the form of daydreams. Our secret longing to love and be loved and our desires for prestige, fame, self-realization, healthy rebellion, wealth and happiness, as well as for sensual satisfaction and erotic ecstasy that have not (yet) been realized gain access to consciousness via this path. Naturally, it would be more liberating if we could stand behind these dreams and surrender ourselves to our positive shadow with abandon and (sensuous) joy.

Favourite jokes

Being humorous means living a "juicy" existence (Lat. humores = juices) that is full of life. With a good sense of humour, life's adversities become easier to bear. At the same time, humor teaches us to not always take everything so seriously and most certainly not ourselves. On top of this, jokes show us that we are not alone with certain shadow topics. The laughter that accompanies them is liberating.

People who have no access to humour, often do not have access to their shadow either. Those who cannot burst out laughing are missing an important safety valve. In effect, they are lacking a discharge mechanism for shadow aspects. As a result, the people concerned get stuck with the highly-charged energy of their shadow.

Contrary to the fears expressed in colloquial sayings, no-one has ever *died with laughter*, nor indeed *laughed themselves to death*. Quite the opposite, the far greater danger lies in *boring oneself to death*. The latter is a very real threat if the persona, with its elaborately-polished masks, keeps life held back behind a well-styled façade and banishes everything that is shadow related by means of repression. This creates a well-ordered, well-behaved, controlled and constrained impression and ends up becoming boring. The life led by the silent majority and that of the (stuffy) citizen in general is not exactly enticing, neither for those concerned, nor for those who are forced to watch the strictly-governed and highly-regulated misery. The possibilities for ensuring release valves show, on the one hand, how much vitality is still there and is still managing to reach the surface, and on the other hand, just how grave and serious the situation already is with regard to the suppression of shadow.

Shadow diary

Are jokes even capable of cheering me up? If so, which ones? If not, why not? Do I no longer even feel like laughing? Let your favourite jokes or those jokes that you like best from the collection provided in the appendix appear in front of your inner eye like little sketches. Try to get a feeling for which topic makes you laugh and shows your shadow. Make a hit parade of your favourite jokes and include the three best ones in your shadow diary. If you consider this order in particular, what does it tell you about the hierarchy of your shadow themes?

Those who are able to roll on the floor with laughter will—in the truest sense of the phrase—be able shake off a few things, that they are then, of course, free of afterwards. In this redeeming way, they can get rid of anything that would otherwise put pressure on and disturb their conservative idyll. In this respect, laughter has a liberating effect, but ultimately also a stabilizing influence on the system. Jokes short- circuit the system and thus enable discharges of energy that are difficult to achieve by other means. If we take a look at various different genres of jokes and select those that we find easiest to laugh at, we will soon discover those shadow areas of our own that are most in need of this kind of discharge. These areas are the ones that are loaded with the greatest tension and reflect how tense we are with regard to this subject. The collection of jokes in the appendix offers you a range of suggestions to choose from. If we find we are not able to laugh at a topic at all and instead react with a stony expression, it could point to a taboo topic and consequently to deep shadow. Only a state of relaxed indifference or a polite laugh show a lack of resonance and thus freedom from shadow.

Favourite books and films

Novels and feature films are an opportunity to take part in the life stories of others. If a certain genre, such as westerns or thrillers, triggers special fascination, this might be an indication of shadow content. William Miller says, "Noting the traits and attitudes of characters with whom we identify can provide an invaluable resource for uncovering our shadow's dimension."[49] It should be added, however, that this identification can be positive or negative. Whether we idolize a character, or a particular role, or decisively reject it, points to light or dark shadow.

1. Those who like adventure novels and war films seem likely to have a shadow problem with the principle of aggression. In this genre, we live out warlike parts of ourselves with the corresponding main actors functioning as our representatives. That

49 Miller, Ibid pg 61

is certainly better than not at all, even though it is also not a real solution. The axis from the unredeemed pole at one end to the redeemed opposite pole at the other runs here from brutal violence to strength and courage.

2. Those who, on the other hand, like novels and films about pleasant country life, which pay homage to down-to-earth values, a firm sense of what constitutes healthy living and basic gratitude for wholesome homegrown food in abundant supply, will surely find shadow in a positive sense here. The axis in this case ranges from oversentimental kitsch in the shadow variant to true enjoyment and pleasure in the redeemed form.

3. In direct contrast, those who are enthusiastic about movies like *Catch me if you Can*, are likely to find their shadow aspects in the domain of communication. The fascination here is nourished at one end by the basic game of hide-and-seek, coupled with deception and disguise, and at the other end, by the uncovering and unmasking of such games. Fans of crime thrillers and murder mysteries, in which hard-nosed commissioners use their superior mental powers to put a stop to criminals, also belong in this category. Their shadow might have to do with cleverness and disguise, and its resolution could range along the spectrum from the gathering and exchange of information through to deep spiritual communion.

4. Family-based stories that emphasise homelife and the natural rhythms of Mother Nature, thereby providing us with a sense of comfort and security, most probably point to a corresponding positive shadow theme in the realm of the archetypically feminine. The unfulfilled longing for these qualities is satisfied by means of books or films, at least for a certain time. A love of nature films could also point in this direction as well. The axis ranges from vicarious satisfaction to genuine cosy nest feelings and sense of community

5. Blockbuster historical epics in book or film form, such as *Troy*, which focuses on a radiant hero shining brightly like the sun, inspire viewers who relate to the corresponding theme of taking centre stage. The axis ranges from the coward hiding in

the shadow to the hero basking in the light.

6. Novels or films about doctors and TV series about hospitals are a genre that is near and dear to the principles of order and good health. The spectrum here ranges from chaos that is being kept hidden in the shadow to true healing in the light.

7. Alongside war and horror flicks, romance novels and films are the most successful genre, which suggests that nothing is as prone to shadow as the themes of love, aggression and shadow in itself. Romantic flicks like *Pretty Woman*, with Julia Roberts and Richard Gere, consistently beat all box-office records and shed light on people's longing for fulfilling love and a happy end, on the one hand, as well as for the ascent from the shadow realm (of prostitution) into the light (of the world of the rich and the beautiful) on the other. Here positive shadow can be seen very clearly. When all is said and done, there is hardly a successful novel or film that doesn't allow the theme of love to flow into it at least in some way.

Shadow diary

What role do feature films and novels play in my life, and what shadow does this show me?

Pick out your favourite genre, and within that, your favourite film or book, and consider them in terms of light and shadow with regard to this topic. Write down in your shadow diary what connects you personally with this topic and this film or book.

You can repeat this for the second and third most important genre.

Which genre do you strictly avoid? Which shadow does this reveal?

8. Thrillers and horror movies betray just how strong our fascination with the darkest of negative shadows is. Why else would anyone voluntarily indulge in the unimaginable atrocities of a film like *Silence of the Lambs* and even pay for the privilege on top of it? The principle of radical transformation also has its own avowed fan base. Its members are, in actual fact, less at

risk of becoming victims of the darkest shadow than those who pride themselves on never watching horror movies of this type. Wild-west themes also belong here, as does the film adaptation of the book *Death Wish*, in which Charles Bronson immortalized the archetype of revenge. Nevetheless, in line with the Law of Polarity, even in the case of revenge, there is still always the opposite pole in the form of good avengers such as Zorro, Ivanhoe and Robin Hood. Fans of maverick detectives, such as the German TV character Commissioner Schimanski, are also being appealed to here. It is their own shadow that is responding when their hero fulfils their desire for justice with lawbreaking deeds and the ability to pack a punch. The spectrum here ranges from the darkest grey to the brightest light and is illuminated further by the myth of the phoenix, which arises from the ashes and ascends to the brightest radiance.

9. Novels and films that convey ethical values, visions, faith and philosophy belong to the principle of finding meaning, and as such, bring us into contact with positive shadow and the deeper sense of our life. A film classic like *Ben Hur* appeals to this form of positive shadow, as does the modern blockbuster *Avatar*, in which a love story is told at the same time. A wonderful film that sheds light on the whole spectrum from deception to true faith healing is *Leap of Faith* with Steve Martin, Debra Winger and Liam Neeson.

10. The medium of film makes it quite difficult to do justice to the principle of reduction to the essentials. Nevertheless, *Broken Silence*, the story of a Swiss Carthusian monk, who is forced to break his silence after many years in order to save his monastery, is one example that belongs in this category.

11. Whacky productions that convey a sense of optimistic new beginnings, such as *Easy Rider* or *Hair*, address the principle of originality and the shadow dreams that are associated with it. The shadow ranges from an anti-social coldness of spirit to glittering and fascinating new worlds of light.

12. The principle of transcendence eludes our world on the surface and thus also the bestseller and film industry.

Nevertheless, in recent times, more and more mystical and spiritual productions have also begun to touch upon this area. This is connected with the search for the unfathomable and profound that is hidden in the depths, with the world beyond our own and our final destination and whose shadow is to be found in the downfall into sectarian and delusional worlds. A beautiful film in this regard is *The Razor's Edge*, based on the novel by Somerset Maugham with Bill Murray.

Choice of career

Just as every profession has its light sides, which are typically emphasized at job interviews and other official occasions, in line with the Law of Polarity, each must also have its dark sides. That the greatest number of arsonists are to be found among firefighters is now a well-known fact, even for those who are not open to the Laws of Fate. In the final analysis, it is also easy to understand. Those who become firefighters want to put out fires. If there are no fires for too long a time, some so-called black sheep become nervous and start to light their own.

The positive job profile of soldiers involves protecting, safeguarding and defending their country. Their shadow is their own insecurity, which can be seen hiding behind puffed-up shoulder pads and medals of honour and can extend all the way to the highly-aggressive displays of power and corresponding abuses of it; it is no coincidence that dictatorial tyrants often end up recruiting themselves from among the ranks of soldiers. The same applies to police officers, who see themselves as our friends and helpers and who are the representatives of law and order. As soon as they start using criminal methods themselves in order to combat crime or allow themselves to be bribed, however, it is the shadow that is sending its regards.

In a similar vein, insurance agents aim to help people feel secure, albeit with bureaucratic means. In actual fact, however, they must initially make people feel insecure and stir up fear in order to drum up business in the first place. An analysis of the shadow reveals how much they ultimately make a living from trading in fear.

Similarly, it is well known how often doctors tend to be afraid of illness in the sense of being hypochondriacs. They constantly deal with these fears in the form of projection onto the patient. When it comes to the light shadow side, a doctor is a healer with a holy and sacred task. In the case of the dark shadow side, however, the doctor is a hypochondriac and an unwholesome scaredy cat, scaring others and spreading fear in turn, and thereby creating an unholy mess, as the last few made-up epidemics and pandemics have made so embarrassingly clear. All those physicians who use scaremongering tactics to force patients into undertaking early detection measures, which they then try to pass off as preventative measures, are also shadow figures, without even realizing it. Eventually, the shadow catches up with them and turns medical professionals into medicynical professionals.

Similarly, it is also naïve to believe that surgeons would generally prefer not to operate if they can avoid it. In this respect, they are far more like the arsonists and tend to operate far too often rather than not often enough. When internal medicine heart specialists examined heart transplant patients after the fact, they found that half of the patients would have managed just fine with conservative therapy. Surgeons have a burning desire to operate, just as firefighters burn to extinguish fires and soldiers to shoot. Everyone enjoys fighting on their own front. It is also good that that is the case, because that is the only way to learn a skill and demonstrate mastery of it in an emergency. Nevertheless, the shadow cannot be overlooked.

When it comes to holistic healing practitioners, their light side is already displayed in the name of their profession. In keeping with this, they practise "holistic healing". In the shadow, however, an "unholy" mess looms instead. For example, in many healing centres, so-called "pre-cancerous cells" are diagnosed more often than truly necessary, only to then be supposedly "healed". Alternatively, the state of the intestinal flora is first ruined in order to then treat it afterwards at great expense.

The more positive the image of a particular profession, the more susceptible it is to tainting and shadow. Several terrible scandals have made it clear that there are a number of nurses who have angels of death lurking in their shadow realm.

That psychiatrists are themselves crazy does not seem like an absurd proposition to most people. In answering journalists' questions about how they were able to put up with living alongside schizophrenics in shared flats, the two great psychiatrists Ronald Laing and Edward Podvoll were at least prepared to admit that they actually felt quite close to the patients and were easily able to relate to them. And in effect, you certainly do have to be fascinated by the tendency of the human psyche to go astray to voluntarily spend half your life and all of your professional life in a psychiatric clinic. Similarly, psychotherapists must be just as enthusiastic about the digression of the human soul and be true shadow fans in order to constantly and gladly accompany people on the aberrant odysseys of their souls. The danger entailed in this, however, can be that they end up working on their own shadow solely in the form of projection, thereby neglecting necessary self-therapy. When it comes to lawyers, it is clear to everyone that they are supposed to apply the law. Nevertheless, as part of their profession, criminal defence lawyers are also required to defend injustice. The saying that "in court and at sea, you are in God's hands" betrays just how unreliable the guild actually is. In many countries in Asia, Africa and Latin America, any such problem in itself is seen as a disruption to the state and bribery is the rule. Obviously, public prosecutors and police officers also need a certain degree of criminal imagination of their own in order to even be able to track down criminals in the first place.

The light shadow side of politicians consists in serving society. An important interim goal in this respect is a ministerial post. The word "minister" means servant (of the state). But instead of serving and leading, it often becomes more a matter of being self-serving and easily misled. Instead of enriching society, self-enrichment threatens from the shadows. The ironic interjection that "those who believe that representatives of the people represent the people probably also believe that forklifts lift forks" is aimed at the shadow of politicians. In order to experience this shadow, it is no longer even necessary to travel to the so-called Third World. In reality, well-known capitals like Brussels and Washington have fallen into the hands of lobbyists on a massive scale that is hard to overlook. Major bribery scandals have also shaken German boardrooms, and leading politicians have often only managed to save their necks from judicial nooses with a great deal of difficulty. The Berlusconis of this world simply change laws before they can be directed against them. Because of this shadow, the population has already chosen to make fun of him by giving him the first name Benito in memory of the dictator Mussolini. Any politician who, like the former German Chancellor Helmut Kohl, accepts large sums of money without being asked to provide a receipt must know that it is black money. Claiming that the noble-minded donors did not expect anything in return is highly naive. If we weren't dealing with the so-called "Chancellor of German Reunification", he probably would have been detained in custody until the names of his cheating friends had been revealed. He only barely managed to get away with it yet again, but with what result? For all he did for Germany on the light shadow side, he also unmasked the dark shadow of politics. The appendix

Shadow diary

Do I have a job or have I found my profession? Does it call to me and is it my calling? What is its light side and its shadow side? Which side do I have more to do with? What am I lacking in my profession and is this the reason why I find myself on the shadow side? Do I balance this out, for example, with a hobby?

Please fill out your shadow diary with your notes.

provides further tips regarding the shadow aspects of various professions, which may serve as a stimulus for a confrontation with your own profession.

(Hobby) Sports

As important as sport is for many people, it may not interest others in the slightest. Should the latter be the case, this chapter and the further tips in the appendix can be skipped—but only after you have become consciously aware of your own sports shadow and interpreted it.

At sports events, the dark shadows of the spectators often become very obvious. For example, they like to sit at the most dangerous bend in a car or ski race, at precisely the point where it becomes particularly life-threatening for the athletes. Sports like boxing, general wrestling or catch-wrestling, where a strong element of showmanship is added, attract spectators because of the openly-displayed aggression. More often than not, the fiery roars, with which their sporting favorites are aggressively rallied on, are even quite brutal and warlike and reveal darkest shadow very directly. Since in these sports, beating and bashing are officially allowed, shadow that is otherwise classified as negative emerges positively and is not only tolerated, but even glorified. "An incredibly strong right hook," notes the reporter, while the boxer on the receiving end of it may suffer the effects of it for life. In ice hockey and football, outbreaks of violence are regarded as calculated risks that occur by accident. The language of the reporters and the battle cries of the armchair experts firing them up, however, make everything clear as far as shadow is concerned.

In the case of athletes, the dark shadow becomes clear in overexaggerated ambition and extreme competition. This is clear, for example, in the openly-displayed joy of a skier when members of his own team are eliminated, in line with the motto: "If not me, then at least none of us". Such malicious joy is the rule in competitive sports, although it is usually not shown quite so blatantly. In women's sports, in particular, sporting shadow is also embodied in figures that are ruined as a matter of course and that are more suited to muscle-packed bodybuilders.

The sport shows in and of itself what has brought it to life and what would otherwise be missing. This in itself is also a shadow aspect. In this way, the type of sport itself indicates what is being sought in life.

The ancient Olympic ideal of the youth of the world meeting for peaceful games, with participation being everything and victory only of secondary importance has long since been forgotten. Sport is a reflection of our highly-competitive performance-based society with its strong potential for addictive behaviour, ranging from our addiction to world records, to top performance and to success. As a result, it is understandable when our highly-competitive, performance-based society promotes highly-competitive, performance-based sport. Even in the amateur and hobby sectors, performance and competition are increasingly becoming the focus of attention, which corresponds to our patriarchal society as a whole.

Shadow diary

Which form of sport did I prefer in the past? Which form do I practise nowadays or which form do I prefer to watch? Which elements does this sport deal with (for example, windsurfing deals with water and air)? In other words, what am I lacking and how do I get it from this sport?

In the appendix on page 259, additional suggestions are listed for your own personal examination of the light and shadow aspects of various professional and hobby sports.

Being at peace with everything

Everything within everything: the holographic worldview

Naturally, and particularly in the beginning, it is more difficult and uncomfortable to recognize yourself as the creator of shadow than as its victim. Nevertheless, there is an old view, formulated by Paracelsus and increasingly supported by modern scientists, which makes this step easier: microcosm equals macrocosm. In accordance with this view, human beings each represent a perfect microcosm in and of themselves while at the same time mirroring the macrocosm that they are a part of. Today, this spiritual theory is much more than a mere model of reality.

The possibility of taking photographs with highly-ordered, so-called laser light led to holography. This method offers the best reflection of the interconnectedness of the world so far. From any part of such a hologram, the whole image can be reconstructed at any time. However, that means nothing more than that everything is contained in everything. This fact has inspired scientists from many different schools of thought and has led to similar statements as those that have been made by spiritual masters. "The drop may sometimes know that it is in the ocean, but rarely does it know that the ocean is within it," says the Indian Yogini Anandamayi Ma. "We are not in the world, the world is within us," explains Ayurvedic doctor Deepak Chopra, whom Debbie Ford quotes in her book *The Dark Side of the Light Chasers*. She herself expresses it even more directly: "We each hold within us a trace of every human character that exists." And Byron Katie once again manages to put it in a nutshell: "Everyone is a mirror image of yourself –your own thinking coming back to you."

This means that, from both a spiritual and scientific point of view, we have everything within us at all times. Therefore, we need not be ashamed of the fact that, in the course of this book, we have also found and hopefully will continue to find a lot of dark, shadowy aspects, but above all, aspects that we were not consciously aware of within ourselves. Ultimately, a further consequence of this is that we can only ever criticize, insult, accuse, condemn or otherwise disparage ourselves. Anyone who realizes this will soon stop such self-recrimination. When it comes down to it, all we are ever really doing is talking to ourselves; all charges brought against others in the form of complaints are actually charges directed against ourselves. Therefore, it is good to at least listen to your own monologues and lectures. Since I have started doing that myself, I have gotten a lot more out of them in any case. And those topics that I obviously find really difficult to grasp are the ones that I am called upon to present very often. From a projection perspective, this would be interpreted as follows: "My book *The Laws of Fate** is obviously very successful because the topic is often requested by event organizers." More honestly and without projection, it should actually be interpreted as follows: "I still don't seem to have grasped the Laws of Fate in all their depth, because I am still called upon to talk about them and over and over again." Richard Bach says in his book *Illusions*: "We teach best what what we most need to learn."

Take a moment to consider whether you don't also often advise others to do what you yourself need to do. We like to remind others of things that we ourselves need to be reminded of, give advice that no one needs more urgently than ourselves. What we repeat most often, what we are most likely to point out, is what we ourselves need most.

Of course, each and every other person around us is not physically within us, but whatever quality is being expressed in their life can definitely also be found in ours. Similarly, while we certainly do not necessarily commit the same deeds as others by any means, we most certainly do possess the same soul qualities that lead to them. In the case of a criminal act, it can help to take a look at the full background story that led to the crime. In this way, it sometimes possible to be more empathetic Additionally, the old Indian proverb, "Never judge another until you have walked a mile in their moccasins" can be helpful, as well as the Christian phrase, "Let him who is without sin among you cast the first stone". As soon as I have found the appropriate trait within myself, I no longer need to be judgemental of it within others.

In the opposite direction, this behavior can be turned into an indicator: in other words, as long as I condemn something, I cannot (yet) have accepted the corresponding quality in myself. This is a wonderfully simple opportunity to develop self-control and practise self-therapy. Whatever I condemn in others is a learning task that I still have to face up to myself.

In the end, the whole thing is very simple: As long as we continue to cast the blame on others, we are continuing to dump the blame on ourselves as well. As long as we are not at peace within ourselves, others will continue to be negatively struck by us. That is why the process of coming clean with ourselves, shedding light on the shadow and living with conscious awareness is worth its weight in gold. Those who find fault with themselves automatically find fault with others as well. For this reason, we need to see the difference between, on the one hand, the necessary process of judging and weighing up alternative options in order to recognize what is (or is not!) of benefit for us, our body, our soul and our spirit, and on the other hand, the process of continually finding fault based on external (judgemental) values. The world acts as a mirror for us. The more we are able to use it to get to know ourselves better, the more aware and the wiser we will become with regard to ourselves and to the world in general.

Those who realize that they have everything in themselves that they see and criticize in others—admittedly not necessarily in exactly the same form, but fundamentally similar—will experience a radical change in their view of the world and their self-image. Based on this, we could learn to simply let ourselves be exactly as we are. Because *everything that we do not let be in us does not let us be and does not let go*. The better we learn this, the easier we can let others be, and our life can then simply unfold. There would be no need for commands or commandments, orders or the controlling of others. The result would not at all be indifference in the sense of a gloomy lack of interest, but instead something that Buddhists call *upekha* or equanimity. Those who can look at the world, their own and any other, in this way, are at rest within themselves and are well-centred. A sense of peace and calmness emanates from them. And, of course, thoe who wants to be at peace with the world must first make peace with themselves. This is what we read in the Tao Te Ching, Verse 57 :

> The more prohibitions you have,
> the less virtuous people will be.
> The more weapons you have,
> the less secure people will be.
> The more subsidies you have,
> the less self-reliant people will be.
> Therefore the Master says:
> I let go of the law,
> and people become honest.

I let go of economics,
and people become prosperous.
I let go of religion,
and people become serene.
I let go of all desire for the common good,
and the good becomes common as grass.[50]

50 *Tao Te Ching*, op. cit.

Meditation

Read Meditations 1 & 15.

Give yourself enough time directly afterwards to let the impressions continue to take effect before allowing them to gradually fade away. Come back to the here and now in the usual way and record your impressions in your Shadow Diary.

Practical Exercise

Consider the ten commandments as offers in the way that they were originally intended. If you follow the ten commandments that are "offered" by our culture, you will produce fewer ugly shadows. You can follow your inner voice, which longs for all that is light and good in the world. The result will be a pure and good conscience, in the sense of inner consciousness, which acts as a proverbial gentle inner cushion of peace.

Psychotherapy, shadow work and the spiritual path

William Miller makes it clear: "Shadow has a life of its own and clamors for attention and time on the stage. Instead of elbowing it back into the wings, and trying to continue to persuade the "audience" that we are only what they see, we need to turn around, face and dialogue with shadow, undesirable as that may be, and gain reflective insight from the encounter."[51]

With this in mind, it should have become even clearer by now why positive thinking never was or can never be shadow therapy. This is because it actually enlarges the shadow by hiding symptoms and whatever is considered unacceptable behind the fortified walls of affirmations. At the same time, the shadow and the ego continue to grow in parallel, a situation that those on the outside have no problem seeing. In addition, as the scientist and author, Bruce Lipton, emphasizes, the affirmations used for this purpose usually only penetrate the upper layer of the subconscious, thereby cementing over the border to the actual realm of the soul, where the greatest treasures lie dormant. In contrast, shadow therapy aims to bring out everything that has been rejected from behind the walls and protective barricades. Debbie Ford says in this regard: "We are told affirmations will make us okay. But as I tell people in my lectures if we put ice cream on top of poop after a few spoonfuls we will taste the poop again. When we integrate negative traits into our selves, we no longer need affirmations because we'll know that we're not worthless and worthy, ugly and beautiful, lazy and conscientious. When we believe we can only one or the other, we continue our internal struggle to only be the right things."[52]

---

51 Miller: *The Golden Shadow*, op. cit., pg 72.
52 Ford: *The Dark Side of the Light Chasers*, op cit. pg 84

Whether we should venture into the shadows on our own or with professional help is difficult to determine with any great certainty. If the shadow has already manifested itself in disease patterns that are affecting the body in a massive way and threatening our very survival, the decision to seek help is naturally more than obvious. However, anything that massively restricts us in life is also a good reason to seek and accept help. Anyone who is planning to follow the life path (of development) anyway could make a lot of things easier for themselves by undertaking shadow therapy[53] as early as possible in keeping with the Gestalt therapist Irving Polster's statement that psychotherapy is far too good to be reserved for the sick. Nevertheless, even after shadow therapy, the game of forming and then resolving shadow continues unabated, albeit on a much more relaxed level and with far better chances of success.

Those who do not feel nearly as hard-pressed by everything can take their own steps into the realm of shadows and will find many tried and tested hints and tips in this book that have proven themselves to be helpful in the lives of the authors and during more than thirty years of shadow therapy at the Heil-Kunde-Zentrum in Johanniskirchen. A first step is also the study of the meditation *Shadow Work** (see footnotes).

As long as we are on this Earth, shadow remains the main topic of interest. Genuine shadow work must clear up all reproaches towards life and the world, this constant blasphemy, and all of our resistance towards Creation exactly as it is. In the context of this main topic, it is important to analyse the totality of all remaining reproaches and forms of resistance in a further exercise.

53 This refers to what is known as Reincarnation Therapy, which is carried out in the Heil-Kunde-Zentrum in Johanniskirchen, and ideally lasts for four weeks (See address in the appendix); See also information provided on the Internet at www.dahlke.at

Meditation

Read Meditations 1 & 16 and give yourself enough time directly afterwards to let the impressions continue to take effect before allowing them to gradually fade away. Afterwards write them down in your shadow diary again.

The finishing touch and the masterstroke

The hardest thing in shadow work is finally admitting to yourself: "Not only am I like this, but I am in fact allowed to be like this"—in other words, not just accepting the shadow but also even loving it. This is the pinnacle and is more rewarding than anything else.

In this highly demanding exercise of accepting and lovingly accepting our own shadow-side, we automatically come up against the Christian ideal of: "Love thy neighbour as thyself". Some people have tried to dodge the dilemma this poses by distorting its essence. All of a sudden, it is turned into: "Love thy neighbour above all else,". In such an endeavour, we are all bound to fail hopelessly and to continue to cultivate a guilty conscience. Those who take Christ and his teachings seriously with regard to this sentence must begin to love themselves in order to have any chance at all with their neighbours. In actual fact, the Master's teachings are much more realistic and easier to put into practice than what was made out of them.

This central Christian principle states very clearly that we should not and cannot love our neighbour more than ourselves. But if we see all people as our neighbours, as is clearly the Christian mission, and want to love them, we must love ourselves completely, and that includes the shadow. Whatever failures occur in this respect, occur at precisely this point. It is only if we accept ourselves as a whole, that is, with our dark sides as well, that we can manage the same with our fellow human beings and their dark sides, too. Only those who embrace and integrate their own shadow, i.e. those who accept and love themselves as they are, can also embrace the shadow of others and accept and love other people just as they are. It is with regard to precisely this point that (almost) everything has failed so far, and as a result, Christianity has ultimately fallen far short of fulfilling its mission, which, as a religion of love, must surely entail spreading this everywhere. Instead of letting love grow from within, the attempt has been made to spread the religion of love by means of the "fire and the sword" in the form of terrifying missions. Christ's mission could not have been misinterpreted any more dramatically. It is by building upon this basis of a Christianity spread by force that capitalism, with its guiding principle of competition, was later able to establish itself worldwide—a consequence that is obviously another shadow phenomenon. Naturally, when dealing with the high aspiration of spreading love, the shadow is particularly powerful.

Wherever we look, we are quickly confronted with the central theme of shadow. If we are serious about shadow integration and want to make progress, we simply cannot avoid accepting and loving ourselves in an all-embracing way. Love and shadow are the solution for almost all our problems to an equal degree and follow the order in which we learn to love the shadow. Nevertheless, that in turn is merely a paraphrase of the overall task of taking back our projections or, in other words, learning to love our enemies.

This brings us to the second central love-related proposition in Christianity. In actuality, we are supposed to not only love our neighbours as ourselves, but also our enemies. In this respect, the theme of shadow reveals itself as a central Christian theme and unites these two main Christian requirements within itself. This book is therefore also a deeply Christian book, even though some clerics have clearly been revealed as shadow figures within it. The light shadow of their dark shadow is that they can still grow—and can do it together with us.

At the end of successful shadow therapy, everything should once again be back in the shop window of life and should be able to be exhibited without shame. Whatever was cleared off the shelves and hidden during childhood and youth is now allowed to appear on display again, regardless of whether it is popular and easy to sell or whether it is not so well appreciated by the public. We appear more natural, more complete and more healed (i.e. more whole) when we also know (and acknowledge) our darker sides and are able to show them. Admittedly, when we initially set off on the path of confronting the shadow, we were most likely afraid of being rejected on the basis of all of the dark aspects of our being. In contrast, we now experience, almost without exception and often full of astonishment, that quite the opposite occurs and growing authenticity and genuineness instead strike a chord with others. Even if certain individual aspects of shadow may be unpopular in themselves, we as a whole come across much better—to ourselves and to others.

When we open ourselves to our shadow, we expand and become more accessible. Our boundaries in relation to others and to the world become more transparent and less perceptible with a tendency to gradually disintegrate altogether. Because we consciously recognize more and more dark sides within ourselves, we become more tolerant towards our fellow human beings and the world and its problems. With the awareness of both sides of reality, we increasingly find ourselves centred in the middle between the two poles. We have gotten to know the extremes and know that, for every pole, there is an opposite pole, and that the truth lies in the middle between these two poles.

In the end, the choice between the two different ways of life, i.e a plain and simple bourgeois life and a holistic, all-encompassing one, boils down to C.G. Jung's famous question: "Do you want to be good or whole? Today a similar sentiment can be found on T-shirts and book titles in the sense of "Good girls go to heaven, bad girls go everywhere". The youth of today obviously wants to follow in Jung's footsteps and go everywhere, although it is unclear whether they are aware of the consequences. In any case, it was clear to Jung that the shadow enriches our lives immensely. He explicitly emphasizes how much its childlike and primitive qualities intensify and add beauty to our lives.

Those who only want to be good necessarily end up owing a great debt to wholeness. Those who want to become whole are certainly allowed to also be good, but on top of that, they can own up to and stand behind their darker and less good sides and acknowledge and love them as well. This makes them more complete and their goodness more genuine and natural. They will not have to defend it and go on the offensive to enforce it as a program for everyone. Instead, they are aware of the other side. It is no longer a shadow for them, for they have directed the light of consciousness towards it, and consequently it belongs to them as well and they are identified with it, too. With regards to other people, they become gentle, recognizing on which level those people currently stand or are wrestling with their shadow. They will no longer judge (and be judgemental), because they know a lot about the darkness in their own shadow realm, and they will be less judgemental, because they can allow both sides to simply be and have the perceptiveness to see the respective significance of each side for the whole. As Krishnamurti taught: "The ability to observe without evaluating is the highest form of intelligence.".

The Angels Program

As long as we struggle in life against shadows in our inner world that we have suppressed and shadows in our outer world that we cannot overlook, we tend to wish our fellow human beings would go to hell, while at the same time, acting like devils ourselves towards them. Since our unconscious shadow is constantly on the rampage, wreaking havoc between the lines in our life, we naturally end up being in resonance with dark energies.

But after we have shed light on the shadow to a large extent and taken possession of our Self, the empty husks of the Persona drop away, and from beneath the various masks, our true Self comes to light instead. From now on, we no longer need to pretend to be someone better and therefore no longer need to pretend to be anyone else either. After all, the attempt to be better than we really are prevents us from becoming what we could be: namely, ourselves. All of that exhausting pretending simply drops away. We are equal to each other, and the exhausting life of competition comes to an end. We are as we are, and we are allowed to be as we are.

Now we have the possibility to become an angel to our environment and to stage positive reversals instead of fulfilling negative expectations. Because these are so surprising, they have the chance to quickly penetrate at a deep level and thereby leave behind a significant impact. An example may serve to show how simply and wonderfully this strategy works:

During a river cruise through Russia, I came across the stand of a young painter at a typical tourist market, offering impressive watercolors for very little money. Upon seeing that I was interested in one, she at once meekly reduced the already small amount even further, apparently used to being pushed down in price by tourists. She spoke a little English, and I offered her an amount for the painting that was significantly above what she had originally asked for. She was even more astonished when I told her that I hoped to now own a picture that would become more and more valuable in the future as a result of her continuing her work. She was deeply touched and astonished, gave me a small green lucky stone and asked for my address. Years later, I received an invitation to her first larger exhibition with a small painted heart. The card said: “Spasibo!”—“Thank you!”

The idea for initiatives of this type had been given to me long before by a German teacher of mine, who had been forced to grade one of my essays much lower because of the many comma mistakes it contained. She said apologetically that the commas were not really important. She hoped she would read about me later, at a time after the commas and school were long gone. I did not understand that correctly at the time, but the comment stayed with me in my conscious awareness. Whether she spurred on my writing I don't really know—just as I am probably not the reason for the artist's exhibition. But perhaps they were each little mosaic pieces in a self-fulfilling pattern. In any case, my joy at the news from Russia was disproportionate to the small extra premium I paid for the painting.

The trick is more than simple: instead of fulfilling negative expectations, turn them around and turn them into a positive surprise! The more shadows we keep hidden within us, the more we will trigger shadow experiences in our fellow human beings. The more shadows we have already shed light on, the easier it is for us to spark light experiences in our fellow human beings—on the one hand, by emphasizing the light sides in their shadowy expectations, on the other hand, by helping to give their dreams a boost. It is exactly these aspects that will stay in our memory for a long time and that will nourish our own soul.

I wish you with all my heart the desire to live your dreams and the strength to shed light on your shadow.

Appendix

Favourite jokes and their shadow

1. Included in the principle of aggression are all jokes leading to sudden outburst of laughter in relation to topics, such as violence and brutality, but also those related to courage and strength.

A man says to a woman: "Shall we? Or would you like to dance first?"

A pickup line of this sort that is so impulsive and brief is typical for the headlong rushing into things and the rash nature of the aggression principle. At the same time, the theme of the opposite pole of love, is already brought into it as well via the pickup line—aggressive flirting, so to speak.

2. The principle of self-esteem, rootedness and sensual pleasure is alluded to in the following:

An ailing, filthy-rich Christian is on his deathbed. His personal physicians have stepped back and his bed is now surrounded by cardinals. In a barely audible voice, the wealthy Christian laments: "Oh, if only I could take my gold ducats with me!" Before the stunned Excellencies have a chance to react, the altar boy blurts out: "Surely they would melt where you're going."

Not only will those who have issues with money and wealth in their shadow feel compelled to laugh, but also those who have banished the finite nature of existence from their consciousness.

3. The archetype of communication is a very popular one for all of us, and in that respect, is enormously widespread and comes into play almost everywhere.

Power blackout in Bonn: Minister Schäuble was eventually freed from an elevator after more than an hour; Chancellor Kohl from an escalator after two hours.

Those who have an issue with intelligence, or those who are conceited or just truly simple-minded, can find relief by laughing here.

Three priests from the same city meet every week for a general chat and the chance to confess their sins to colleagues: After a while, they begin to trust each other more and more. The first one says: "I hardly dare to say it, but I've already taken money from the collection plate." The second one says: "I've already used collection-plate money to spend a nice weekend with a sister from the parish." The third one says: "You won't believe it, but I suffer from a compulsive urge to gossip and can't wait to spread the news."

The people who laugh here are those who have "Schadenfreude" (malicious joy at the misfortune of others) in their shadow and who themselves are not averse to gossip.

A Jesuit and a Franciscan are sitting on a train and reading their breviaries when the Jesuit lights up a cigarette. "But Brother, surely this is forbidden," the Franciscan says to him. "No," the Jesuit replies, "I have special permission from the Holy See". In disbelief, the Franciscan takes it upon himself to investigate the matter further and promptly receives the expected negative response. At the next meeting, he bursts out with righteous anger and accuses the Jesuit straight to his face... "Brother, you are a liar." The latter replies: "Oh, I forgot; you're a Franciscan. You probably asked if you are allowed to smoke while reading your breviary."—"Of course!" replies the Franciscan. "You should have asked the other way round whether you are allowed to read your breviary while smoking."

The people who are inclined to smile here are those who are like to make use of manipulative and cunning tricks themselves without always be willing to admit to it.

4. All those who hold the deep-seated fear that they are not intelligent and clever enough for this sophisticated world; all those who instead believe that they appear rather naive, simple-minded and perhaps even stupid; all those who have not yet discovered their own natural rhythm and are not yet able to proudly stand behind their femininely-soft, maternal tendencies are the ones who are most likely to laugh the most at blonde jokes, since such jokes suggest that there are others who are obviously worse off in these respects.

Question: Why do blondes keep empty bottles in the fridge?

Answer: Because there are some guests who don't want anything to drink.

Blonde jokes target starry-eyed naiveté and femininity in general. At the same time a lack of intelligence is hinted at, for example, in jokes of the following type:

Question: Why do blondes hold their hands tightly over their ears?

Answer: Because they're desperately trying to "hold that thought".

5. The following joke addresses the archetype of the center of attention from the opposite pole.

> *At a meeting of the three conductors Böhm, Bernstein and Karajan, the first of the three says: "Dear colleagues, it has now even appeared in black and white in the newspaper: "Karl Böhm, the greatest living conductor". Surprised, Bernstein replies: "Karl, just last night, God himself said to me in a dream: "Leonard, you are the greatest conductor of all times." Smiling, Karajan asks: "Sorry Leonard, what was it you think I said to you last night?"*

Those who laugh heartily in this case most probably have their own delusions of grandeur and need to be the centre of attention hiding in their shadow and will find these reflected in pretentiousness and the corresponding megalomania of this kind. This allows the pent-up tension behind such unacknowledged pretensions to be released in a fun way. Many of us have unacknowledged ideas of great magnitude and a corresponding fear of our own genius and excellence, as well of the power of their grandeur and the force of their energy. In jokes, this fear can be spontaneously release herself and thus create relief.

6. Those who in post-war Germany got a laugh out of the HB-guy, a hapless cartoon character with a short fuse, which was used to advertise HB cigarettes, were not only making use of the opportunity to gloat over someone else's misfortunes. The poor little guy desperately fought against various trials and tribulations of the post-war economic boom with no hope of success. Everything went wrong for him, and those who also had things go wrong for them, albeit not as many things, could laugh their heads off. On top of that, there was a dash of cynicism in all of this, because each of these unfortunate episodes ended with an image of the HB guy smoking the appropriate cigarette and a voiceover of the saying: "Enjoy with a happy heart—then everything will work itself out". In view of the risk of heart attack,

which for precisely this kind of person is considerably increased by smoking, this was too much and the advertising slogan had to be withdrawn.

Nowadays, it is TV shows with hidden cameras, which cater to this topic instead and allow millions of viewers to enjoy the misfortunes of their fellow citizens that are sometimes truly horrific. Clips showing the bloopers and mess-ups of professional presenters and speakers are a source of amusement for the average citizen, who doesn't really get much out of them and certainly not any access to their own shadow. Here are some further jokes related to this principle, which is also connected with "craft and tinkering", as well as organizing, health and nutrition:

"Do you believe in astrology?"
"No, not really. We Virgos are very skeptical people!"

On a luxury cruise liner, it is time for dinner, but rough seas avail. The waiter finds his guests moaning, as they hang over the railing, green with seasickness. With great sensitiveness, he asks: "Should I serve dinner first or would you rather I simply tip it overboard right away?"

The doctor reports: "Colonel, unfortunately, you have gonorrhea.
"I must have caught it on the toilet," he replies.
"Oh, how uncomfortable!", the doctor says.

When someone once said to Voltaire, a notorious smoker, that tobacco is man's greatest enemy, he replied with a smile: "Certainly, but don't forget that we have been told that we should love our enemies!

7. The domain of love and beauty, peace, reconciliation and partnership is of great concern and is a challenge for us, and is

therefore full of shadow. As such, it provides ample material for jokes. The following joke, which is almost identical to the one told in the Aggression Principle, also fits the relationship counterpart of aesthetics and love:

He: "Shall we go to my place or yours?"
She: "If it's that complicated from the start, let's just forget about it."

Sexually-suggestive stories make up a good portion of the jokes. Of course, there is the well-known saying that "Dogs that bark, don't bite." In a similar vein, those who tell lewd and dirty jokes all the time, may need that outlet because they don't have another one. They could see through the (shadow) game at this point. It may also be that someone has long since stopped being able to laugh at these kinds of topics. This would also be a clue worth following in the search for shadows.

8. The particularly-challenging principle of radical change comes to discharge in the genre of "But mommy…" jokes:

"But mommy, I want to skip," the daughter whines.
"No, Daddy has to stay hanging until the police arrive!" complains the mother.

Those who can laugh at macabre jokes have accumulated shadow in the area of radical metamorphosis, which then gets aired through this channel:

"Bin Laden Airlines: We fly you directly to the office!"

Jokes that make you laugh at the totally absurd also belong in this domain:

Three carp are sitting in a cellar shooting the breeze. "Goal!" shouts one of them, "Checkmate" says the other.

Those who unconsciously fear that they don't really have it all together can lift their spirits here.

9. Jokes cloaked in religious guise and dealing with questions of philosophical beliefs fit the principle related to finding meaning in life:

An old Jewish man is desperately banging his head on the bench and complaining to Yahweh: "My son has turned away from his faith and converted to Christianity!" Suddenly, the heavens open and God's powerful voice booms down from above: "Tell me about it!"

The vicar, who is filling in for the priest for confession, asks the altar boy "What does the priest give for anal intercourse?" The boy answers: "One Mars bar and two Snickers."

The bishop paces up and down in front of the altar, striking his chest and mumbling to himself: "I am nothing, I am nothing." The priest sees this and does the same. The parish clerk follows suit. The bishop then turns to the priest and says, "Look who's already trying to be a nothing!"

Those who laugh or smile at this will have shadow problems with self-aggrandizement and hubris.

10. The following joke reflects the principle of reduction to the essential:

After a long search, a seeker of truth finally finds the revered sage in a simple little room, furnished only with a chair, table and bed. Dismayed, he asks "Why do you have so little?" The sage replies, "You yourself have even less." "Yes," says the seeker of truth, and justifies this by adding, "But I'm just passing through," The sage responds wisely. "You see, I am too,".

Those who can laugh or at least smile here might have shadow problems with simplicity and reduction to the essential.

11. In principle (archetypically speaking), jokes belong to the principle of originality, as they revolve around both sudden moments of craziness and spontaneous discharges of energy. Consequently, every joke with an unexpected punch line that sparks laughter could serve as an example here. Incidentally, those who happen to live only for jokes have their shadow here; their whole life ends up becoming a joke.

At our place, everyone is called Karl, except for Fritz, who is called Franz.

Here, bewilderment and confusion are given an outlet.

The pastor on Sunday says to his congregation: "Dear Christians, the sermon is cancelled today, because I actually have something to tell you. "

To be is to do—Lao-Tzu. To do is to be—Sartre. Do be do be do—Sinatra.

In Bavaria. a church tower gets hit by lightning and burns down. The following Sunday, the pastor asks for donations for the reconstruction works. Farmer Binder say: "Well, Reverend, I'm not willing to give a dime to a landlord who sets fire to his own house!

The great guru had no sense of humour. For this reason, he became the butt of countless jokes. Outraged, he asked one of the ringleaders responsible for the spread of the jokes: "Did you make the joke about me and the pig? The person concerned couldn't deny it. The guru replied: "How dare you make such jokes about me, the only fully awakened and enlightened master on this planet? The ringleader felt the need to protest: "Hang on a minute, you can't blame that last joke you just told on me!"

Last of all, the principle of the dissolving of boundaries brings up the rear for our jokes, which do not find particularly fertile ground in relation to this topic

A patient visits a psychotherapist and complains: "Doctor, I am always being overlooked." —"Next, please."

Different professions and their shadow side

1. In professions that are dominated by the principle of aggression and new beginnings, for example, in the military domain (soldiers) or the medical field (surgeons, dentists), the positive light sides of the principle in the form of courage and strength, high energy and decisiveness are required. The dark shadow aspects loom in the form of audacity and recklessness, foolhardiness, assaulting others and abusing power.

2. A profession related to the principle of self-esteem, rootedness and sensual pleasure is, for example, that of the restauranteur. On the light side, there is a commitment to nourishment, service and replenishment. On the shadow side, serving others can potentially turn into exploitation and taking them for a ride.

Cooks are the modern-day alchemists and conjure up new recipes to transform food in ways designed to make it more digestible. In doing so, they are supposed to prepare these food items in a healthier way so as to ensure our enjoyment and well-being. In this respect, they are supposed to lay the groundwork for the female principle of care and nourishment. More and more often, however, they see themselves as artists—and are supported in this belief by television executives. This leads them to produce so-called "delicacies" that are scarcely worthy of the name. In French cuisine, they serve perversities such as foie gras (i.e. pate made from the liver of a duck or goose that was fattened up by being force-fed grain), frogs' legs and lobster, and in Japanese cuisine, the list includes fish that are still breathing and the brains of monkeys that are eaten while they are still alive. The resultant shadow from this is food that, far from being very digestible, instead aims at sensationalism, while losing sight of the health aspects.[54]

Waiters have humbleness and the desire to serve as their light side, but all those who have been purposely ignored know their shadow side in keeping with the motto "Watch out, there's a customer threatening to make an order".

3. Journalists are (over)active in the field of exchange and communication. As seekers of the truth, they are naturally obliged to inform and educate. But how often do they lay it on so thick with their truths that the breaking headlines tend to be crushing for others instead. Manipulation and twisting the truth, disinformation and fear-mongering, but also the spreading of gossip and lies are the shadow aspects here. "Our newspaper was the first to speak with the deceased": this parody of a headline reflects this shadow quite well.

In the teaching profession, the shadow issues are an inability to accept advice or criticism from others and slow-wittedness. Teachers tend to treat everyone like children and repeat even the simplest things again and again like a mantra. Friends speak of a high level of redundancy and are referring to this love of repetition. Those who mainly deal with people who are less educated and intellectually (still) inferior, might be able to discern the rather arrogant shadow pattern of the chronic know-it-all, as caricatured in the stereotype of the German schoolmaster. Lecturers who impart knowledge also belong here. On the one

54 My book Weight Problems* lists the various shadow aspects connected with different types of food and particular national cuisines.

hand, their shadow is revealed when they become so caught up in the specific details of their subject that they degenerate into blinkered specialist nerds. Alternatively, they could also use their knowledge to manipulate others and exercise power. In general, they should master life themselves and put theory at the service of practical life, instead of constantly lecturing others

4. With regard to the principle of *sensibility, emotion, sense of security, and rhythm of life*, well-paid professions are scarce, and yet this is one of the domains that people work the hardest in. Housewives and mothers convey security, cosiness and understanding. Their shadow is neglecting themselves. They are afraid of loneliness and of not having any roots of their own, which is often expressed in chronically cold feet. Often the desire for contact is more play-acted than real, which is reflected in cold hands as well. Shadow also becomes clear when strings are pulled behind the scenes, with conditions being set between the lines and under the radar. Manipulation of this is carried out and demands such as these are made, so that the children live out the wishes of their mother in their profession and choose their partner with her eyes.

This fourth principle also includes cottage industries, other work-from-home jobs and the nursing professions. Nursing others to the point of self-abandonment has the helper syndrome in its shadow, as well as a great need for recognition and reward. The shadow can also extend to unwanted euthanasia. In this case, the lowly humility necessary for this profession turns instead into the haughty arrogance of raising oneself to the position of being lord and master over life and death. Even more shadow is involved if the ulterior motive of legacy hunting was behind their actions.

5. The principle of creativity, charisma and centredness includes the profession of manager, which is exercised by people who tend to be the centre of attention, and to lead others while always being in the lead themselves. The term "Chief Executive Officer", which is nowadays commonly shortened to "CEO", already includes the military term "officer". As such, it calls to

mind the concepts of leading and fighting, as well as the conquering and taking over of markets and shares. The shadow lies in the potential for *mis*leading and *self*-enrichment, as recent headlines have made clear. Rather than ensuring that their own company was the centre of attention and leading it to the pinnacle of power, quite a lot of them ended up sidelining themselves instead, along with their company, which in turn provoked book titles like "Nieten in Nadelstreifen" (i.e. Losers in Pinstripes).

Artists actually belong in the realm of aesthetics, but nowadays, many people no longer want to be artists, but instead aspire to be instant stars. As such, they belong to this principle of being the centre of attention and its corresponding shadow. The light side becomes clear in their function as role models; the shadow side becomes apparent in the corresponding negative image of such idols that is increasingly coming to light with regard to airs and graces, drugs, violence and other forms of (im) morality. The term 'art' was originally applied to great skill and craftmanship and later took on the additional meaning of an aptitude for scholarship. Nowadays, however it is not uncommon for art to instead mutate into "W-art", where the simple Wish to achieve something overshadows the actual ability to do so.

6. In addition to the aforementioned physicians, the principle embodying *order and reason* also includes pharmacists. On the light side, they are responsible for developing and blending together remedies and miracle cures. In their shadow lies the making of poisonous concoctions. In this respect, the pharmaceutical industry also has its own broad shadow, which exacts a high toll. According to conservative estimates, thousands die each year as a result of their remedies. In Germany alone, the number is thought to be about 17,000 patients.

7. Obviously, confectioners and bakers, who decorate their sweet creations in a wonderful way and bring us closer to the sweetness of life with their seductive treats and snacks, of course, belong in the sweet kingdom of the principle of *harmony, relationship and aesthetics*. In the meantime, however,

the shadow in the form of Type-2 diabetes has begun to take on epidemic proportions.

Goldsmiths and jewellers refine and enhance beautiful things with their creativity. That this may lead to a discrepancy between appearance and genuine substance represents a danger for their customers. As for themselves, shadow could also show up in the form of using non-precious or perhaps even fake materials and charging unreasonably high prices.

Of course, in this wonderful domain, there are also true shadow professions, such as the brothel madam, pimps and professional dating services. Their shadow reveals the light aspects of eroticism and love.

8. The professions associated with the realm of *radical transformation* can be found in the domain of shadow therapy. Stuntmen, who continually put their life on the line for money also belong here. In their case, it is more the light side that is in shadow. They could end up getting killed and experience the greatest transformation possible.

9. Priests and missionaries are committed to their faith and thus to the principle of *growth and finding deeper meaning*. Representing God on Earth in a dignified way is their task, playing Him as a role their curse, and threatening people with the fear of hell and thereby making a pact with the devil their shadow-filled everyday business. The "ground crew" of many religions has become the incarnated shadow of the original intentions of the respective founder of the religion involved. Muhammad wanted to help and serve women and to lighten what, back then, was an even more difficult load. Anyone who considers the (over) zealous mullahs and their attitude towards the feminine today automatically feels the chilly breath of the shadow. Christ bestowed the religion of love and forgiveness upon us, and his representatives have caused rivers of blood to flow in his name.

10. Civil servants are committed to the state, its continued existence and well-being, and thus to the principle of *structure and reduction to the essential*. However, with such a large bureaucratic apparatus of civil servants, it is hard not to gain the

impression that, as a result of the ever greater proliferation of bureaucracy, they have begun to devour their state, or more accurately, to bleed it dry. The apparatchik and the bureaucrat in their respective opposing economic systems prevailed long enough until one of the two systems perished as a result and the other is, at the very least, showing signs of also suffering serious damage. Although they were signed up to ensure order, they are instead responsible for the idling mode and chaos that bureaucracy causes, and sometimes their sheer numbers alone seem to lead to them becoming the gravediggers of their respective states.

11. In the domain of *independence and originality*, there are a rare number of professions. Here one could think of inventors who make life easier and better with their innovations. However, most patents collect dust in drawers because they do not serve this light side, but instead correspond to the madness of their inventors. The dark side of many inventions today cannot be overlooked. The light bulb shed light on the world while at the same causing an energy disaster. The introduction of its successor—the energy-saving lamp—was perhaps well-intentioned, but has turned into not only an aesthetic disaster, but also an even greater ecological one, as well as on top of all of that, being a health problem.

The auto(mobile) initially made us more mobile and is now increasingly leading us into traffic jams and other states of standstill. It could therefore be said that it has been "overtaken" by its shadow. While the individual models are getting faster and faster, they are making slower and slower progress on the roads as a whole. Politicians all over the world are making themselves the extended arm of this shadow by restricting their mobility and free travel even further.

12. The *border dissolving* principle not only involves mystics and meditation teachers, but often also actors and not uncommonly bankers, who are supposed to ensure the free flow of money. On the light side, their task is to ensure that money—as a medium of exchange—remains available and in circulation,

thus making production and projects possible. However, since the last great financial crisis, the shadow has caught up with them. Instead of providing people with money and keeping the economy going, far too many bankers massively enriched themselves by playing the stock market, eventually plunging the economy into serious stagnation and crisis.

Shadow topics that are vented in sport

Without claiming to be exhaustive, the following is a list of largely popular and widespread sports that apply to many and thus address important shadow areas, such as those of aggression, instinctive drives, ecstasy and the lightness of being.

Ecstasy

Sports that are capable of inducing ecstasy include wind and wave surfing, kitesurfing, dancing and horseback riding, but also alpine skiing and sailing.

In the case of skiing, the fascination most probably lies in the high speed and the direct contact with the air element, whereas in deep snow, the free, almost weightless gliding and letting oneself drift at high altitudes is also added to the mix. Passionate deep-snow skiers are seeking such feelings and could learn to let them flow into other areas of their life, such as the domains of eroticism and love, with benefits for their development. The direct shadow of their longing comes into play when they get stuck standing in lift lines on their skis.

Windsurfers hold the wind—that child of heaven—in their hands and dance over the waves. At the exit point of a power jibe, the increase in speed becomes palpable, the body lighter, and this gives rise to a feeling of lift-off—the lightness of being becomes tangible. The surfers grow wings in the form of the sail, and they hang in their trapeze—floating quite freely—between the sky and the sea. Spectacular catapult crashes reveal the shadow of this.

Wave-surfing brings speed and the challenging danger of the devouring, archetypally-female water element into the game of life and can in this way convey feelings of ecstasy. In the past, surfers were not interested in competition, but instead simply in a pure, flowing attitude to life.

Kite surfing or kite boarding combines the water and air elements in an even more elemental way. Like Icarus, his followers have wings and use these to rise above the world. Their kite, like a flying dragon, imparts the thrill of flying and the lightness of being. Paragliding can also bestow this feeling, as can sailing over the ocean waves, which allow windsurfers and very light boats to experience a gliding sensation.

Glider pilots also float on waves of air, and of course most pilots share this dream as well. They lack lightness in normal life, and the bouyant feeling of soaring above it all has probably been lost in the shadows. It is revived on such sporting occasions, which is why quite a few athletes only feel truly alive in such moments. "Life is surfing, the rest is details", was written on a poster in the office of a manager, who held a leading position and was also a family man.

Sky-diving (both the free-falling and hovering phases), as well as for a select few, ski jumping and ski flying also belong in this category. Most of us tend to prefer watching the latter as spectator sports and ro enjoy the sensation of flying from the safe position of projection onto our heroes.

With dancing—from the Viennese waltz to the dhikr, the ritual whirling dance of the dervishes—it is also about ecstasy. Here it is particularly easy to detach the astral body from the physical body and to experience the accompanying feeling of bouyant, floating lightness. Ultimately, all forms of dance, if they have been appropriately mastered and are then enjoyed freely, are a reflection of life as a dance. In both cases, one ideally submits to the rhythm and lets oneself be carried along, probably setting one's own accents, but always in harmony with the pattern of the music. The gruelling work of professional dancers that quite literally grinds them to the bone reveals a dark shadow aspect of this career path.

Equestrian athletes find their happiness on this earth on horseback, especially if they are free of competitive ambition and allow themselves to simply surrender to the interplay of forces. Anyone who more or less soars above the horse rather than bearing down on the saddle when galloping at full speed over long distances, who gallops freely over wide open beaches or rushes through splashing water, may have the feeling of experiencing themselves as God intended. Whether it is light snow or loose desert sand that splashes to the side under drumming hooves, the rhythm of a galloping horse can change one's own (life) rhythm for a few enchanting moments, elevating it to new heights and bestowing a feeling of heart-pounding liveliness. Against the background of the above-mentioned sports, you can try answering the following questions for yourself: *Where do I live my right to ecstasy expressly? And how does it feel? If I don't live it expressly, but stow it away in the shadows, where could I live it out? Which sport could most likely help me to feel ecstatic? Who or what hinders me from doing that? How do things stand at the moment when it comes to sensual ecstasy?*

Building up stamina

As the opposite pole to ecstasy-inducing sports, it is also worth mentioning workout rituals, such as jogging, cross-country skiing, swimming and other endurance sports. Here it is often good health that is the focus of attention. Movement is undertaken in the so-called "oxygen equilibrium" zone[55], not only to do the organism good, but also the soul. When endurance sports are engaged in just for fun, it is most probably about finding

55 See All Good Things Come in Threes*

one's own rhythm and managing to keep going in order to develop (greater) stamina. Those concerned develop toughness, persistence and resilience. In addition to generating good health and vitality, these characteristics are bound to nourish whatever they aspire to and thus represent positive shadow.

When it comes to mountain climbing, the path of life and how to master it is added to the mix: ascent and descent parallel the different phases of life; there is also the intense sensation of being close to nature, as well as the exhilarating and sometimes truly ecstatic experience of reaching the summit. Whether the mountaineers realize it or not, when seen from God's perspective, every tour to the summit is the path through the mandala:[56] i.e. from the periphery to the centre and back again.

Cycling also belongs to the category of endurance sports and, like every sporting discipline, has its own symbolism, which clearly reveals the shadow component involved: Here someone is choosing to stoop voluntarily. As such, this sport is the caricature of a frequently-seen attitude to life—"bootlicking the bigwigs while trampling all over those below". No wonder cycling is the most popular mass sport, at least in Austria.

Running, or "jogging", as it now called even in German, also reveals certain shadow aspects. In connection with this, it is worth asking ourselves whether we are running on the spot (on a treadmill) and not getting anywhere or whether we are constantly running round in circles following the same daily rout(in) e. It is also interesting to be aware of whether we are running over sticks and stones or soft-and-springy forest ground or subjecting our joints to the assault of an asphalt surface.

Shadow questions when it comes to powerwalking or Nordic walking are: *Do I actually know how to do this properly, or am I simply carrying two sticks around and looking a little strange? Am I in a bit of a rush? Am I already using a walking stick?*

As far as athletic disciplines are concerned, the shadow questions are particularly easy to find. For example*: Do I always go*

56 See The Workbook on Mandala Therapy*

round and round in circles on the stadium track like a hamster in its wheel?

In the case of long-distance and marathon running: *Am I training my capacity to keep going until I can't go on any longer?* After all, the historical predecessor of this sport used to lead to death due to overexertion and utter exhaustion, and as we now know, of course, how things start is how they tend to continue. Obviously, all of that was still not enough for our overambitious, performance-driven age, and in the meantime, even more extreme excesses, such as the sport of triathlon have arisen—with no regard for the consequences and that demand a big heart on the wrong level.

A look at the 100-metre sprint necessarily begs the question: *Do I always have to be the fastest?*

For decathlon, the question is: *Do I really need to become the king of all athletes?*

Jumping competitions are obviously all about *getting the (right) amount of thrust*; the corresponding heroes are always *on the go*: long jumpers aim to make the greatest leap forward while high jumpers set their sights high.

Those in the throwing disciplines like to *push things forward* and go far with them, in the same way that as all of us, when it really comes down to it, also want to go far, too. Some hurl a hammer like the Germanic god Thor, others Odin's spear, some throw shotputs as though from cannons, and many feel like sporting hotshots, at least in a figurative sense.

Questions that arise with regard to this division of sport are: *How do things stand at the moment with my stamina? My ability to stay the course? What am I doing to develop this further? And is that enough for me? Should I perhaps make timely use of Nordic walking sticks before Fate forces me to make use of a different kind of walking stick? Or should I get moving in a different way? And on what level?*

Training for our life path

The aspect of our life path is symbolically expressed in many sports, such as (competitive) skiing. Our potential energy decreases with every meter of altitude, and as is the case on our lifepath, obstacles are placed in our way that need to be hurdled, steered clear of and overcome—from bumps to jumps to slalom poles. Despite having a certain amount of individual freedom to find the ideal trail and approach in life, the overall course is by and large predetermined. It is important not to get stuck and to not end up straddling the poles, to adapt one's speed to the terrain and the circumstances and to reconcile the need for safety with ambition. It doesn't matter whether people are competing professionally or at an amateur level, because amateurs also enjoy speed and, depending on their nature, will try to push themselves to the limit or even go beyond their limits.

In the case of waterskiing, you dodge buoys instead of poles and the jumps are always man-made; the only difference is that the energy source is a motor(-boat) instead of the slope.

Perhaps the theme of following our path in life is most evident in a sport such as orienteering, which admittedly tends to strike a chord with far fewer people comparatively speaking.

In order to track down the shadow, it would be worth asking: *How could I practice tracing my path through life? Find the ideal course? The red thread? How do I deal with obstacles on the way? Do I try to confront or go around them? Do I dodge life or front up to it?*

Sport and energy

In some sports, such as motor sports, the fundamental energy involved comes from the outside world, as a gift, so to speak.

Those who feel attracted to such sports actually come to expect this energy as a gift and enjoy playing with it.

As such, they are completely different to those who like to torture themselves at marathon or even triathlon events and put their Ironman, man of steel or "Iron John" qualities on display. In such events, the aim is to show that nothing can kill them; that this particular man, or even woman, is as tough as steel and is not afraid of even the worst of ordeals. These kind of people enjoy working hard and want to truly earn everything they get by themselves. In line with this, they tend to be lean and gaunt in appearance.

For sportsmen who rely on an energy supply from outside themselves, as in car or motorcycle racing, this aspect of working to serve is mostly lacking. Horse-riders also like to be given energetic gifts. In this respect, the difference between alpine skiers and cross-country skiers is, of course, also very clear.

The question to ask is: *Do I prefer to play with energy that comes as a gift from the external world? Or do I enjoy building up energy within myself and then later expending it?*

Martial arts

Whether we're talking about western variants, such as boxing and wrestling, or eastern ones from tai-chi to karate, the ultimate goal is to work on the principle of aggression in ritual form, and in the best case scenario, to redeem it. Even the western martial arts variants also prescribe a strict ritual framework to do justice to this principle, which is generally considered dangerous. Probably due to the principle of aggression, the announcer in boxing typically tends to be a screamer, who gets paid a lot of money to scream the names of the fist-fighters into the microphone in a dramatically- exaggerated and ridiculous way.

Most sports inherently contain at least some components of Mars energy. Even chess is about attack and defence and about capturing and defeating the opponent. Even the different forms of defence are still aggressive.

- Ask yourself: *Do I recognize and use sporting rituals as a chance to reconcile myself with my aggressive energy? Where else do I allow my aggression to come out? What do I get out of these rituals and what do I do with it?*

Games

Games betray a desire for playfulness. Here it could be a matter of getting an inner child that has been left behind in the shadows back into the game of life again in a fun way. Fast-moving reactive games, such as tennis or even more clearly, table tennis or squash, add a time component. Doing the right thing at every moment and very quickly is the order of the day and is the only way to succeed. Whether someone plays table tennis or gambles on the day-to-day fluctuations of the stock exchange is, in this respect, pretty much the same. It is all about the longing to be in the right place at the right time and to do the right thing. That is, of course, also the secret of every successful life.

The (archetypal male) goal of most games is to dominate the field, outplay the opponent and knock them out of the game. This demonstrates their lack of control of their own field, on the one hand, and their inability to endanger the successful aggressor in their own field on the other. All the while, the latter continues to encroach on their field at will and to lord power over them. In the process, the cards are reshuffled at every moment, which forces people to be truly present in the moment. As a result, it is necessary to play every point and to remain focused at all times. A marathon run, in contrast, is a comparatively long-winded, routine affair and is tied to a completely different topic.

Defending one's own territory, attacking that of an opponent, making sure one's own goal is protected, capturing the goal of the opponent—from chess to football, these are the old patterns of war that hopefully will be able to replace more and more real wars. "Football World Cups instead of World Wars" is the wonderful name of the game and shows the shadow component of this truly world-shaking sport. In this sense, sport has an extremely important function in maintaining (world) peace and as a form of shadow therapy. Fortunately, for all of us, many more people nowadays work on their shadow aspects—on the sportsfield instead of on the battlefield, and sportsgrounds are also much more heavily occupied than therapy rooms. At the same time, these different settings are by no means mutually exclusive. Many political battles have been fought on sportsfields since the 1936 Olympic Games and especially during the Cold War. And, of course, as I have the pleasure to experience personally, it would also be possible to combine psychotherapy and sports in order to live up to the ancient ideal of "*Mens sana in corpore sano*" ("A healthy mind in a healthy body").

Group games, such as football, handball, volleyball and water polo, show our longing for clan and community, for team and family. The different positions are based on real life, starting from the basic polarity of defence versus attack. Here we could ask how team-oriented or selfish our own game is. Or how we react as a spectator to egotistical actions as opposed to selfless actions. How did you feel about the popular school game of dodgeball, where the aim was to shoot down as many opponents as possible in order to wipe out the those who were on "the other side"?

Ask yourself: *What games do I like to play? And at what level? Do I play along, or do I want to shape and determine the outcome of the game? What do I like about watching games? What do I never watch? And what does that tell me about my shadow? Am I interested in the community aspect, or am I still a lone fighter even when in a group? How beneficial to the group and selfless or maybe even selfish is my game? How well is my inner child doing in the game of my life?*

Football as a popular sport

A sport that people all over the world engage in and find so stirring must also span worldwide shadow aspects. This operates not only at the level of the sport as a ritualized substitute for war, and as an outlet for nationalism; it is also a means of identification for people with a weak self-image. For many, the (football) club becomes a substitute home; the national team becomes everything that is important and valuable for them, and consequently, the (national) coach rises to the role of a better dad. Rarely do they agree with him—in actual fact, only when the heroes of their own family win under his guidance—but they are forced to follow him nevertheless. He is allowed to decide everything, for example, when the eleven (millionaire) boys have to go to bed and whether they are allowed to bring their girlfriends with them (to training camp or what is actually more like a youth camp). They hang on his every word and discuss his decisions with like-minded people. If he leads the boys to victory, he is the greatest; if he doesn't manage to do so over a longer period of time, he needs to be sent packing. This then becomes a matter of national importance and necessity. All of this is about ritualized battles and consequently the principle of aggression. Most of the reporting that takes place makes use of the language of war; the increasing propensity of players and fans to resort to violence and their growing unfairness make corresponding shadows clear. When the battle groups of the so-called "hooligans", the modern-day visiting (war) spectators, go into battle, battalions of police arm themselves and face up to them resolutely. Often, the battle for the various city centres rages for hours.

As a fan or active sportsman, ask yourself: *What turns me on in football? What do I react to? Do I have a club that I suffer alongside, go into battle with and whose triumphs I share (vicariously)? What does this act as a substitute for in my life? Do I have a special football idol? What position does this person play? And what does that tell me? Do I play myself and if so, in which position? What does football give me? Which longings am I giving expression to, which fears and aggressions? And what do I give to the sport of football in terms of time, money and overall life attitude? Which of my own longings and fears become clear from my preferred playing position? Have I found the ideal position in football for me? Have I found the right playing position for myself in life? Which of my shadow aspects does football make clear?*

The individual positions on the field represent differ functions in life that all need to be mastered. In football, they are neatly arranged in a clear manner. What I play or prefer to play here will either come easy to me or be missing in my life, depending on what I use the game for—to shine or to compensate. The difficulties I may have with it reflect those I have in my life as well.

In the daily life struggle, as in football, defence is the order of the day. The most prototypical of defenders is the goalkeeper. Within his field of influence, he is allowed to do pretty much everything to "keep his nest clean". He's the only one permitted to use his hands in football. His duties include low-risk, safe manoeuvres that he uses to keep the backs of his fellow teammates covered. In his case, spectacular moves are more likely to seem suspicious, as they suggest either mistakes made by the players ahead of him or his own.

By definition, defenders play a defensive role. Instead of ingenuity, sturdiness and a consciousness for playing it safe are required. They need a clear overview and to be considerate of their goalkeeper. A special position is held by the libero, or so-called sweeper, who has to answer for the mistakes of others. He is the only one in the defence who—as a free man—can contribute new input. He needs an even better overview and always has to be in the right place at the right time. Ideally, he should also provide the impulse to move forward and the new game structure should originate from him. Since things tend to continue as they began, the (previous) game stands and falls with him. He is also able to nail the ingenious passes that bridge the space, and in the best case scenario, open it up, which are otherwise typically the responsibility of the midfield. In the midfield, it's all about making connections, bridging gaps, and setting up the game by means of decisive passes that open up the (opponent's) space.

Strikers stand for the actual goal of the game, which is to kick goals and score points. They are the executioners in the language of war and the ones who get the job done in the language of everyday life. There are many different types among them: clever artists and dribblers who outplay and outmanoeuvre their opponents, but also breakers who barrel their way through the middle using power and force and therefore like to act as centre-forwards. In their (war) reports, commentators, often use the term "storm tanks" without thinking of this as being too military.

Ask yourself a few basic questions about all of this: *How well do I fill out the various individual positions in the football game of my life? The role of the goalkeeper, the defender, the libero, the midfielder, the striker and the finisher? Where are my shadow issues and my aspirations in these respects?*

How can I make the most of the learning opportunities offered by football? What about my ability to be a teamplayer? Am I at all interested in teamwork? Can I align myself with pre-assigned patterns? Can I grasp a given role and carry it out in its essence?

In those free spaces that I successfully fight to open up for myself, do I manage move beyond them ? Can I increase my powers of integration even more? Increase my ability to push through obstacles? Can I improve my love of orderliness and my overall sense of how things are distributed within space?

How can I train my resoluteness? Strengthen my capacity to keep my nerves at bay, for example when the penalty kick is "one for all"? Can I follow plan and deploy a particular tactic?

Is unselfishness within my capabilities? Can I learn to put my ego aside? Are fairness and fair play important to me in my life? Can I subordinate myself to a greater goal? Do I stand by Sepp Herberger's motto: "You need to be eleven friends", or do I have no problem with the modern hype around particular stars, which tends to drown out team spirit? Can I subordinate myself to the idea that we want to become number one, or is it more important to me to be number one myself in individual reviews?

Motor control and the mastery of instinctual drives in the case of riding

Ultimately, riding is all about the mastery of instinctual drives. The horse between one's thighs, as a symbol of instinctual drives, needs to be mastered. Young girls who are approaching puberty are often ardent admirers, not so much of equestrian sports as such, but of individual horses and spend a lot of their time doting on them with loving care. For many, this yearning immediately diminishes when boys enter the pubertal game of life.

As the name implies, in military riding, it is militancy, and thus, the rough and manly aspects that come to the fore. This is where the most serious accidents in equestrian sport occur. It is not unusual for horses and riders to come to serious harm; tough guys and girls who are not afraid of death and who are willing to ride through thick and thin feel attracted to this branch of the sport. At the same time, there is also dressage involved, which shows that, even in military riding, discipline and rhythm are also necessary.

Show jumping symbolizes giving one's instincts a jumpstart and aiming to reach great heights in life. In actual fact, the horse is an animal that prefers to flee and not a jumper at all; unless its life is danger and it is panicked, it tends to go around obstacles instead. The rider must therefore push the horse into a comparable emotional state and then still manage to master it. What for a long time was considered a sign of masculinity and thus also a typically-male sport, has in recent times, in keeping with the spirit of the times, also known female winners. Women and men have always competed against each other in the same field.

In symbolical terms, dressage equates to forcing instinctual drives into submission with an archetypally-female tender hand and the unification of obedience and beauty, and rhythm and style with power. In the same way as there are more male elements overall in show jumping, there seem likely to be more female elements and winners in dressage. Here one would have to ask what it means to act as a man in a more archetypally-female discipline, and of course, vice versa.

In Western riding, there has been an amazing reversal of values. Whereas, in the past, the Wild West used to be really wild and often brutal with horses, Western riding now involves responding in a particularly sensitive way to the horse, and as such represents moving from the "New World" into the old one that always was more sensitive in the first place. Nowadays, it is all about having empathy with the nature of the horse and showing it the way, first and foremost without violence. The modern "cow"-boy, which has always been a thoroughly female symbol, is now living up to his name. From horse whispering to show jumping without a snaffle, more and more sensitive and intuitive ways of riding have been spreading lately, showing the need for these sensitive, archetypally-female elements in equestrian sport.

The question is: Do I feel attracted to riding?—Do I ride myself? Or do I like to see it at tournaments or in Wild West movies? What fascinates me about it? What does it say about me, and which of my shadow aspects come to the surface and out into the open in this respect? If I would never go riding, why not? What scares me about it and is therefore lying in the shadow realm for me?

Sporting shadow questions

- Which elements does my particular sport bring into my life? Air—as in the case with paragliding, hang-gliding, ski flying or on the trampoline? Water—as in (dolphin) swimming and diving; Fire—as in boxing and dancing; Earth—as in weightlifting and shot-putting?
- How does my sport affect the body in the long run? What I strive for as an athlete is part of my positive shadow.

Are muscles or even mountains of muscle being built up, as in bodybuilding, and is it therefore a matter of (raw) strength or rather of speed-strength, which instead emphasises the speed of performance?

- Is acute peak performance being aimed for or more endurance? Is it a matter of flexibility or of stamina?
- Is the ultimate goal of my efforts the classical brawny athlete modelled on Hercules or the lean and willowy beanpole instead? Or am I aiming for the emaciated endurance hero of the Clemens Forrell character in the "As Far as my Feet Will Carry me" film?
- Does the emphasis lie on being an all-rounder with a broad range or on high performance in a small specialized domain?
- Is the sport a way of testing my limits, in order to expand or overcome them, of experiencing new spheres, or instead of feeling confident and strong in familiar terrain?

Gender-specific aspects and symbolism in sport

In keeping with the emancipatory spirit of the times, typically-male and typically-female role patterns are progressively vanishing. Nevertheless, many sports can still tell us something about gender roles. Boxing and wrestling continue to be largely male domains and are likely to attract people for whom masculinity is a shadow topic. This also applies for karate and many other Mars-driven martial arts, but also for ski jumping. Soccer and rowing are only secondarily a matter for men and are increasingly being conquered by women. However, as can be seen from the development of the body and figure over time, these also lean in an archetypally-male direction.

In contrast, typically-female sports, such as gymnastics and synchronized swimming, remain completely closed to men, although there would probably be little demand for them anyway. This shows that there are many more women still trying to conquer male domains than there are men trying to conquer female domains, which may have something to do with the corresponding shadow related to power in our societies.

Most types of sport lead men deeper into their archetypes, whereas women often end up following male patterns, as the examples of shot put and javelin throwing show. A pair of Russian sisters, Irina and Tamara Press, who were very successful in both disciplines, were referred to as "the Press-brothers", and unfortunately lived up to this name in terms of their appearance.

The relative value placed on Yin and Yang in society is also shown in the fact that only the leading sports in the male pole are highly regarded. Typically-female sports, such as dancing, gymnastics, synchronized swimming or ice dancing fail to strike a chord or gain recognition in a patriarchal society.

The female pole also eludes objective evaluation and measurement and, in a society that wants to measure and evaluate everything objectively, is thus already suspect. Admittedly, aesthetics and grace can be assessed by means of giving marks, but this procedure is particularly at the mercy of self-serving manipulation. There are only very few typically-male sports, such as ski jumping and sometimes boxing, that have such elements aimed at subjective evaluation.

Just how great the role of symbolism in sport is, is shown by the example of golf. Although in principle the sport is just as accessible for women, the symbolic pattern behind it is so masculine that they feel little attraction to it. Few women would ruin their relationship or company for golf. But men do it time and time again, and in no other sport, to such an extent. At the same time, golfing is ineffective in terms of building muscles and not very good for improving physical fitness—a great sportsman once said that it was about as demanding as picking your nose. Nevertheless, it still fascinates men to an enormous degree. Getting the small ball into the small hole as quickly as possible, without complication and without frills is a typically-male preference and is something that women are familiar with on other levels and that they tend to frown upon. Quite the contrary, they love the diversions and embellishments, the various types of play associated with the game and the close calls. Getting it in the hole directly is a familiar source of vexation to them. Why would they feel attracted to such a game? In fact, among the many women golfers, many of them may have started playing merely for the sake of their husband. Some of them probably only chose the golf course as a way of being able to go for a walk with him in an inconspicuous manner, because he was simply too grumpy on other walking paths and promenades.

The direct hole-in-one in golf, throwing the opponent to the mat in judo or flat on his back in wrestling, finding the crucial gap in the defences as quickly as possible in order to score in a straightforward and effective manner, getting the opponent on the ropes during boxing, quickly knocking the stuffing out of him, and while he is still panting and moaning, delivering the knockout mercy punch—all these are highlights of male-focused (sports) performance that neither turn women on nor encourage them to imitate them—on any level.

In motor sports, the archetypally-male symbolism of potency comes through particularly loudly and clearly. The howl of 400 HP under their right foot or in the right hand turns men on who dream of great potency and who have the corresponding shadow topic. For women and men without the corresponding dysfunction, this is all too loud and too embarrassing. Having the power at hand to instantly go from zero to a hundred amid a thunderous roar is only necessary for those who otherwise are not progressing in life as quickly as they would like. In this respect, the amount of horsepower under the hood often reflects compensatory efforts regarding impaired potency in the pants department—a shadow topic that is particularly unpleasant for men. The drivers of the respective fireballs are often troubled by a considerable amount of shadow that has developed. However, trying to talk to them about it rarely leads to greater realization and awareness. Instead, it often triggers destructive expressions of the underlying aggression problems that frequently go along with this.

In order to round off the sports topic, you can try answering the following questions: *How much masculinity and how much femininity do I experience in sports? And do I do so in an active or passive way? What symbolism is expressed in my sport? Which symbolism becomes clear to me if I now review my sport in my mind's eye?*

Meditations

1. INTRODUCTORY RELAXATION

Lie or sit down in a quiet and peaceful place
where you can be completely by yourself
without any interruptions.

And if you haven't done so already, now is the time to consciously close your eyes.

And no matter what the place that you have chosen for yourself is like,
you can now allow the ideal place for a journey such as this
into the realm of shadow to gradually emerge before your mind's eye.

A place where the coming ritual of discovery
can unfold in the best possible manner,
where everything is ideally suited for this step that is to be taken and that will best support and encourage your willingness to move forward in this way.

And as all of these thoughts are crossing your mind, the most fitting place is already developing further and continuing to take shape in your mind's eye.

And it is always the first thought that rises to the surface that will move you forward

and that is now helping to build up your landscape even further in this special place

for this ritual of shadow integration.

And, in this way, you can perhaps already experience now or maybe even sooner

how everything fits together in a strangely wonderful way

so that you can already see more and more clearly how you are in the centre of this place

and how all of the forces of Fate

are on your side,

as they are always on the side of

development and growth.

And in this way you are already experiencing

how everything around you is coming together

for this special moment,

with every further visit to this unique inner place, it will appear more and more quickly, and more and more clearly, in your mind's eye,

and wrap you safely within its special atmosphere.

And already, you are probably now experiencing an increasing sense of relaxation and growing calmness in the depths of your soul >

inspirational ideas and thoughts are rising to the surface on the gentle vibrations of your breath>

you're sinking even deeper and letting go>

is becoming easier and smoother as the journey continues perhaps even deeper than you originally thought possible >

you're being led by inner images and ideas accompanying you on your way into the depths of your own world of soul images >
is where the journey is heading as if by itself>
from the first rising thought, others are developing, with this ritual place becoming ever more safe and dependable, >
you're now making your way to yourself to experience your deepest depths >
is the reason you have come here allowing yourself to drift into this special moment,>
your breathing is becoming calmer and deeper, the rhythm carries you forward, is life, and life
and breathing are one.

And your inbreath and outbreath join together
as each exhalation allows you to let go more deeply and more easily,
so you perhaps already feel how you can let yourself fall, and becoming calmer,
land more and more in your centre
as the connected breathing carries you safely,
breath by breath, bringing more and more life energy into your body,
so that you can perhaps already feel how the rhythm of breathing out and in,
of giving and taking is a gift to you,
and connects you with the life energy Prana, which, by breathing in a connected way, you can perhaps already sense
as a slight or increased tingling or vibrating or whatever else under your skin, or on it or wherever.

And this connection to the flow of this life energy may seem new to you at first and now ever more familiar and pleasant, or soon, when you allow the gentle flow of this connected breathing to carry you further to yourself and your sense of purpose and being, and with each inhalation, you not only take in air and oxygen, but also Prana life energy. And this may even intensify the feeling of aliveness. And now, with every inbreath, you can already begin to think of a smile, your smile, and in this way, breathe in the expansiveness and openness of this smiling attitude towards life and allow it to fill up your lungs so that they spread out like two inner wings. And you may already feel, perhaps very consciously, that you do actually have wings, these inner wings, your lungs, which you are now actively stretching out with every in-breath and expanding as far as possible to bring in energy and vitality, while you let yourself sink even deeper, allowing yourself to be carried along further with every out-breath, and allowing your smile to pour itself into the space in between the inner wings of your lungs, the heart space. With each breath you take in, your heart fills up more and more with the expansiveness and openness of your smile. And you now think only about your heart and your smile and experience how your heart can actually smile in its own, heart-felt way, and perhaps, the middle of your chest is already filling with warmth, with a certain softness, so that you are beginning to enjoy this special smile that is coming from your heart. And you can now already compare it with the smile on your face, which has probably originated from the depths of your eyes, spreading out from them slowly and warmly all over your face, allowing it to radiate with expansiveness and openness, even though your eyelids are closed.

And perhaps the smile of your heart will now seem even warmer than the upper, almost heavenly smile of your eyes, or maybe the smile of your eyes will appear even more radiant and more expansive. Or soon, as your breathing flows gently, bringing in new smiling energy with every breath you take in, you can allow yourself to sink even deeper with each outbreath you let go of and you can allow the smiling stream of your out-breath to spread the expansiveness and the openness into your outstretched lungs and your heart space, flowing all the way down to your belly, providing warmth and softness, and certainly awareness, down there as well, and carrying the smiling energy down with it so that the belly, in its own belly-like way, also starts to smile and a further belly-like smile begins to develop while you sink even deeper. Breathing out is now already so natural and in flow>,

the smile in your belly intensifies and finds its own form of expression. And you feel how, accompanied by words and sounds, you now glide ever deeper into relaxation to your centre and it is already becoming clear to you how silence and calm can move and trigger even more in you.

When you compare your belly's smile with the smile of your heart, you may already begin to notice the difference, or soon, when you let go even more and entrust yourself to the moment, here and now, it will become much easier and much simpler. You can almost feel how the warm smile in your centre has a different quality than the one from the belly down here and the upper, heavenly one in your eyes. Now, in the depths of both eyes, at its source, you can feel this smiling energy also flowing inwards and experience how both sides of your head and both halves of your brain are also beginning to smile. You can sense its expansiveness and openness as you sink into your centre, and you will feel more and more at home in this ritual of reconciliation with your shadow and feel better with every further visit on this level. And you can already sense how the coming moments of sinking deeper, and especially of silence, will lead you to deeper and deeper insights. And every thought that rises first to the surface can quickly and lastingly imprint itself on you in this deep state of relaxation, and as quickly as it emerges, can take root and provide clarity.

2. AT ONE WITH EVERYTHING

And now, go to a moment in your life where you felt one with everything and you were happy.

Take the first and most impressive experience that rises to the surface and relive it now in inner images and sensations, in the silence that is now spreading out around you.

And if no such experience shows up, just imagine what it will be like when you feel at one with everything and are happy.

The silence will give you enough space for that. Give yourself the time you need.

3. DO I WANT TO BECOME HEALED & WHOLE?

And now, while you are in the depths of relaxation, take the time to let some important questions arise, which will find answers in the first thought that floats to the surface.

Do I really want to become healed and whole and to make peace with myself and the world?

What if I were to live the vision I have for my life as the Aborigines—the people from the origin as the name suggests, originally did?

Could I really let go of my symptoms and problems and become healthy? Or is the secondary gain from my illness far too great?

What if I just gave up pretending and became honest?

What could happen if I accepted the lies that I have been telling myself and the world as lies and let them go?

What would happen if I gave up my frequent "carry-on" and the rest of my criticisms of reality?

What if I started to simply live with what is?

What would happen if I gave up my best justifications and excuses?

What if I stopped repressing my reality in an attempt to find ever new rationalizations?

What would happen if I simply gave up my perfectionism, which for so long has been leading to problems of self-esteem instead of to a state of completeness?

What if I instead accepted my two sides, and those of all other people and things in this world. What if at this moment I stopped resisting what is in my life, no matter what it is?

What would happen if I used all the energy released in this way for self-development?

And what could happen to me if I dared to take the often very small steps that lead to massive results?

Take your time in the coming silence to allow these questions and the answers to really sink in and to consider which ones are still open?

4. WHAT ARE MY ENEMIES MIRRORING FOR ME?

And now allow yourself to take in the following questions and let your soul answer with the first thought that comes to mind.

When, where and in what ways do I actually show the qualities that I dislike, criticize and condemn in others?

What do my enemies and adversaries mirror about myself?

Start with the first person who immediately springs to mind in your thoughts.

Which of my own characteristics that I find most unpleasant do I experience in which people?

The coming silence now offers you enough scope to face up to further thoughts in this direction, to work through other enemies and adversaries and to look into other unpleasant qualities.

5. WHAT DOES MY

ENVIRONMENT TELL ME ABOUT MYSELF?

And now, take the time to ask yourself the following questions and note the corresponding first thoughts that rise to the surface.

If the world is a reflection of ourselves, what does mine say about me.

What does my environment look like at the moment?
And what does that say about me?

What is my current environment mirroring for me about the situation I am now in?

Take the coming silence as an opportunity to go even deeper and to extract corresponding thoughts from these questions and their answers.

6. BLAME AND RESPONSIBILITY

And now consider your own style of shifting blame and responsibility to circumstances and things.

And then note the most important situation in this respect, which will now emerge with the first thought that comes to the surface, and also consider it noteworthy.

Immerse yourself in these circumstances and try to sense intuitively what their essential nature is.

And with each thought that first surfaces, recognize what its basic and inherent essence involves.

7. WHAT WAS MY POSITION IN THE FAMILY?

And now allow yourself to take in the following questions and give the first thoughts that rise to the surface the chance give you crucial answers.

What was my position in the family?

And what shadow did that cast?

As the baby of the family, I will probably have developed fewer leadership qualities than the oldest.

Which topics were taboo in my family?

And each time, we are only interested in the spontaneous first thoughts that come to mind about each question?

How did my parents deal with aggression, with energy in general?

How much power did they have and did they exercise it?

Were they capable of making decisions and tackling challenges courageously?

Or was cowardice a shadow topic for us?

What was your parents' attitude towards sensuality and sexuality?

How was solidarity dealt with?

How did we communicate within the family?
How openly or covertly was information exchanged?

What role did a cosy atmosphere play, how uncomfortable or extremely comfortable was it in our home?

Did our life have warmth and rhythm?

Was it a nice nest and did I like coming home to it?

How much space were we allowed to take up for ourselves?
And how much space did I take up?

How much attention and recognition did I get?

What was our focus? And what was at the fringes? And what was beyond the periphery in the shadow realm?

How were my fears dealt with?

What role did communal fears play for the whole family?

How hygienic was our life, or perhaps even, how sterile?

How beautiful was my home?

How harmoniously did my parents treat each other?

Were aesthetics important to them?

And what was the harmony of the family members among each other like? What role did it play?

Were death and the finiteness of life an acceptable topic or were they taboo?

What role did getting to the roots of new developments in a radical way play?

Was there openness for great changes and transformations?

How much courage and civil courage was there in my family in severe crisis situations?

What role did religion play?
Was it about "religio" in the sense of reconnection to the original source or was it more about church visits?

Did my parents have a vision that they passed on to me? Did they perhaps even have a vision for me?

Did they promote my own vision and support me in it? Or did the whole topic of the meaning of life hardly ever come up?

What role did order and structure play in my parental home? Both on a small scale, in my childhood bedroom, and in the world at large?

Which values determined my parents' lives? Which ones slipped through the cracks?

Was there room for boundless creativity and even craziness?

Did my parents allow themselves to get carried away and to get out of line every now and then?

Was I also allowed to do that sometimes, or perhaps even often, or never at all? Or was conformity a topic of theirs?

Was the mystery of life a talking point for them? Did they have a mystical streak or were they fascinated by mysterious and otherworldly things? Or was there someone else who was in their place?

Did they give me a connection to the unfathomable, to the miracle of life itself and of my life, or did everything remain strictly rational?

If, in retrospect, I use my parents as a mirror, what limitations did they impose upon themselves throughout their lives? Which restrictions did they in turn impose and pass on to me as well?

But above all, what did they not pass on? What slipped between the cracks and is now still lurking in the shadow?

Use the following silence to allow these connections to yourself to truly sink in.

8. CHILDHOOD

And now ask yourself the following questions and always trust the first thought that rises to the surface.

Did a kindergarten play a role in my life? What did it imprint upon me? Was the kindergarten, and consequently also me led religiously?

Was there any particular philosophy propagated there?

And what traces did it leave behind in me?

What was not allowed at all, and therefore ended up in the shadows? What was considered desirable and what was required?

Was I part of a group, a clique?

Which does this group mirror to me retrospectively?

What was important in our group?

What was out of the question at all, and thus directly in shadow?

What role did I play in this circle?

Which position did I have?

What fell by the wayside as a result and ended up in the shadows?

What role did my most important friend play?

What characterized our friendship at that time? What has endured to this day?

What was not allowed to be at all and is therefore still in the shadow today?

What kind of general high school and maybe even advanced secondary college did I attend?

What was their influence on me?

What was taught to me especially thoroughly there? Aand what was recommended to me for later life?

And what definitely ended up in the shadows in any case?

Did my school education have a specialization? What ended up in the shadows as a result?

What overarching values dominated my education?

Which values did not play a role at all and ended up in the shadows?

How did my education make an impression on my life through its very nature and the atmosphere associated with it?

What came up too short?

When and in what way did television infiltrate my life?

Which role does it now play timewise for me?

What else has been overshadowed by this, for example, in the way of personal chats and discussions, cosy gatherings, and my own creativity?

When did the computer enter into my life?

Has it dominated my life since then and has it pushed other aspects into the shadows, or is it leading its own shadow existence?

What significance did my parents' relationship have for me?

Whatever they swept under the carpet has also ended up there for me as well.

Which of the relationship patterns of my parents am I repeating?

Where am I doing precisely the opposite?

Which shadow aspects put a strain on my relationships?

In what ways do they suffer?

What are the distinguishing features of my friendships nowadays? Do I have a close male or female friend that I can discuss everything with, and whose position in relationship to me allows them to address even dark shadow issues?

What characterises my relationships to my colleagues and business partners?

Which topics are avoided, are taboo?

Which shadows result from this?

What is taboo for me and us in terms of money and material possessions?

Do I possess my money or am I possessed by it?

Have I had enough of it in both senses of the expression?

Is it enough to realize my dreams in material terms?

Or have I had enough of this whole topic and am constantly getting hung up on it?

What significance does politics have for me? What can the political issues and the people involved that upset me tell about my shadow?

Do I still get involved or have I simply become resigned?

What do I project onto politicians and onto which ones, and what does it say about me?

Do I have something like a personal philosophy of life?

Which shadows does that entail?

What vision does it offer?

What aspects of this tend to slip through the cracks and into the shadow?

How much independence do I live out in the different spheres of life in my relationship? In my job, and in raising my children? On holiday? In the running of the house? Financially?

What role does personal responsibility play in my life?

With whose eyes did I choose my partner?
With mine, or those of my parents?

Did my choice of career come from the heart, or where did it come from instead?

Did I choose my favourite subjects and hobbies myself, or who else was involved?
And what hasn't come into play to this day?

What role does my nationality play for me?
What arrogance and feelings of guilt result from this?
To what degree am I smug, or how much do I suffer from the fact that I am Austrian, Swiss, German or a different nationality?
And which nations have slipped into which shadow roles?
Are these perhaps wandering around like gypsies somewhere in my unconscious, or am I bending things to fit that perhaps do not correspond to my reality?

9. HILLSIDE VIEW OVER A FLOWERBED

And now, having reached a state of even deeper relaxation, imagine yourself looking down from the top of a small hill onto a huge flower bed. Here you can see the topic that you have remembered from your negative list, however terrible it may be, expressed symbolically, and in a very concrete way, in the form of a floral pattern. This appears so clearly before your mind's eye at this precise moment that it becomes quite unmistakable.

Immediately take note of the first thought that rises to the surface and consider it noteworthy. The terrible aspect that you have remembered from your list will, of course, lose some of its shock value in this flowery form. And, as a result, you may be able to play around with it to find its inherent gift quality or at least to have an inkling of it. And with this picture, you can now go on a journey through time. And imagine and experience in fast motion how summer is progressing more and more rapidly and how it is swiftly changing into autumn. The flowers wilt before your mind's eye in record time and their blossoms turn into seeds. And you now join the interplay of energy yourself and concentrate all of your magical mental powers on this field. And as winter is gradually laying its white shroud over the flowerbed, you experience in thought images how the energies in the depths are rearranging themselves and how the powers of imagery and effect are forming something new from the old energy. You can probably already guess what is now coming. Next spring, from the seeds and the energy of these same flowers and this same topic, a regenerated pattern that fits you even better will grow into a redeeming message that will set you free.

And just as you think of this, and driven by the great power of this special moment, everything starts to grow in the newly-emerging spring season. And in your mind's eye, this presents itself ever more as a gift to you in the blossoming flowers in symbolic or concrete form. As the flowers blossom again in fast motion, the message is revealed to you in this fascinating, flowery way. And at this moment, you may already recognize this as a personal gift to you that you have earned through your efforts on your life journey so far. Completely in the here and now and open to this gift from the depths of your soul, you may already appreciate how, coming from the realm of shadow and the earth below, it reveals itself ever more clearly to you. In this way, it can become flesh and blood and thus second nature to you. And as you continue to recognize it more clearly and deeply, all of this increasingly makes sense to you. This is so much more than a beautiful floral gift. Instead, it is a gift that you have worked hard for and literally earned by making the journey to yourself so as to be able to serve your purpose in life. And, naturally, your gift will spontaneously imprint itself on your mind in its symbolic form. You can now freely welcome it into your heart with a smiling sensation: And then, in the coming silence, allow this experience to sink even deeper and to resonate in the world of your soul imagery and thereby understand clearly to what extent this re-polarisation will change your life. And when you later come back to the surface, it would be best if you could also represent the new symbol in your shadow diary, either in writing or by drawing, and place it on your negative list in all its positive splendour next to the original negative concept. And now take your time to let all of this gradually sink in deeper before re-emerging.

10. MY PERSONAL HOUSE

And now, in this state of deep meditation, ask yourself the question of what your own, very personal home looks like.

Has it become a real shadow palace over the years?

Or is it still an expansive house full of light just like in childhood?

Close your eyes, and with the first emerging thought, let your house appear in front of your mind's eye on your inner canvas.

The first thought that rises to the surface will help you until you have your whole house with all the trimmings in front of you.

And now take a look into the various rooms, the ones that are still full of life, as well as the ones that have been quasi sealed off over time due to neglect and disuse.

Take a mental picture of each room, and now perhaps even one from its light side and one from of its shadow side.

And commit each one very deeply to your memory.

The coming silence will help you to do this, and as you sink even deeper, you will experience even more and make even more significant discoveries. It does not matter whether you find four, seven, ten or all twelve rooms, simply take your time.

11. SUB- AND SPLIT PERSONALITIES

And now allow yourself to very consciously engage with all the sub- and split personalities in your life and ask yourself very directly, "What mixture of divisive elements have I invited into my life?

Imagine a meeting with all the subtenants of your psyche and consciously go to that party. Your party, where you are a guest in the role of your various sub-personalities.

The opportunity to get to know them all in this way, your sub-personalities, does not mean that you will be rid of them, but if you make their acquaintance now and become familiar with them, you can, in the future, rise to the position of usher and direct each of these divisive elements to their rightful place.

In this way, you can grant them the space they need, on the one hand, but you can also control and make use of their energy on the other.

Have some fun getting to know each of these trouble-free or troublesome types and forceful or over-pushy ladies.

And now, whenever you get to know a new visitor at your party, recognize or experience him or her alongside of you and within yourself.

The coming peace and quiet will give you the ideal opportunity to make so many of these crucial acquaintances in your life.

12. DREAM HOLIDAY

And now, take the time to relax and imagine your next dream holiday, where everything truly fits to you in an ideal way.

Use this moment of peace and quiet to allow your own holiday paradise to take shape before your mind's eye. And again, it is the first thought that comes to mind that will help you further.

And while these impressions of your dream holiday are still sinking in, you can now imagine your ideal partner and allow that thought to develop as well.

Let this man or woman of your dreams take shape in front of mind's inner eye, trusting as always the first thought that arises.

13. VISUALISING A FANTASY CREATURE

And in this state of deep relaxation, it will now be possible for you to spontaneously visualize your inner boarhound or inner demon. This will be the first dog or the first mythical creature that has already appeared in front of your mind's eye or that will soon do so.

And now in your internal world of soul imagery, go for a long walk with your inner boarhound and get to know it so well that you can keep it on a short leash in the future and in doing so have it much better under control.

This inner demon will remain with you for a while longer, until you can allow all of its energy to flow into more productive areas. In the peace and quiet that is to come, you can prepare yourself for how this could happen in an ideal way. Ask yourself as well, which gift you could use to tame it effectively.

And since this is a shadow figure, it naturally also has a gift for you. Find out now which one, and continue to enjoy this special walk in silence.

14. WHAT DO I STILL FEEL RESISTANCE

TOWARDS?

And now ask yourself, “What else do I feel still resistance to?” and the first thought that emerges will help you to clarify this question.

What resistance am I definitely not willing to give up?

What resistance is vital to my survival, or in other words, to the survival of my ego?

Where do I still consciously or even intentionally offer resistance?

And in what domains does it happen more or less unconsciously?

And now use the silence to make peace with this deepest resistance of yours.

15. ADVICE THAT I GIVE TO OTHERS

And now, in this deep state of relaxation, turn your awareness inwards and recognize what you most commonly and most frequently give others advice on.

The same advice would most certainly do you a lot of good as well.

Those who constantly scold their children about tidying their room may want to scold themselves as well about tidying up their life, and putting their living space in order.

And what topics are you constantly asked to give advice on?

And what does that tell you? What advice do you give yourself when you give advice to others?

And what do you like to remind others about so often and so gladly?

Is it something you want to be reminded of yourself or something you should you be able to remember yourself?

What do you repeat most often?

Where would you need it most yourself?

Where do you most need to and want to let go of things as your top priority?

What gets in the way of you or how do you get in the way of allowing yourself to let go?

Use the coming silence to find even more in-depth answers to these questions.

16. ANY FURTHER REPROACHES?

And now ask yourself, "Do I still have any reproaches left in me? Any further complaints against anyone or anything?

If so, am I still dealing with shadow? Which particular shadow is involved?

Where do I still feel disadvantaged and dissatisfied?

Which negative feelings are still poisoning me? And turning my heart into a den of thieves?

What am I still hiding from others and what am I hiding from myself?

Am I leading a secret double life? Do I have a hidden story?

Which mask am I still hiding behind?

And how are things with my level of gratitude towards life and the fullness of creation?

And what has my shadow taught me so far?

And to what extent can I already feel grateful towards it at this point?

How much energy have I already gained from it so far and how much can I still gain from it in the future?

The coming restful state will give you the opportunity to pursue these questions and to express your gratitude.

www.ingramcontent.com/pod-product-compliance
Lightning Source LLC
Chambersburg PA
CBHW011744020426
42333CB00022B/2712

* 9 7 8 1 5 9 1 8 1 3 4 6 0 *